the teaching of TALKING

What Other People are Saying

Throughout the pages of this book, we introduce the revolutionary concepts of *The Teaching of Talking* method. Here, we would like to share what people who have been trained in and used these concepts are saying about it.

Testimonials from Patients

"Mark is responsible for me speaking again." **M. Peterson**

"What an amazing human being! He's very caring, funny, responsible, patient, compassionate, understands the needs of his patients, wouldn't quit. He works so hard to accomplish one goal, and that's to help the person talk again. But best of all, he's a friend — a wonderful speech therapist, but an incredible friend — for believing in me. Thank you, Mark." **M. Gutierrez**

"Mark Ittleman has been taking care of my son, who had severe speech problems after a stroke. With Mark's therapy he has made remarkable progress and has learned to communicate reasonably well. I am grateful for Mark's accomplishments and his success with my son. I especially like and appreciate Mark's humor and cheerfulness and rapport he established." **E. Liebenthal**

"Mark provided excellent diagnosis and guidance as I worked through my swallowing issues. Mark is easy to talk to and is approachable and supportive." **J. Francis**

"Dearest Mark, A token of our appreciation of everything you have done for our mother, Great #1 Therapist! We are so blessed to have you! Today is one year from the time of our Mom's heart attack and stroke! She has come a long way from no speaking to talking! You're the best." **Teiko, Scott, Debbie and "Coco"** xoxoxoxoxo Love, xoxo

"Mark's compassionate response to my husband was wonderful. His patience in teaching him to embrace language again has made a huge difference. Mark's understanding of the need to utilize everyday actions and activities in developing my husband's speech abilities was a blessing from God. Because my husband could utilize the lessons immediately, he worked harder and looked forward to each session. Of all the therapies my husband has experienced in five years at -------this has been one of the best due in large measure to Mark's caring, respectful, engaging nature." **C. Welch**

"Mark is always positive and understanding. He is innovative in his approach to treatment. He truly understands my needs and through his vast experience has challenged me to continue. I look forward to my therapy sessions as they are both challenging and supportive. Mark has been an inspiration to me." **M. Doucette**

Testimonials from Supervisors

"To whom it may concern:

"I have had the pleasure of knowing and working with Mr. Mark Ittleman for almost two years as his manager at an outpatient rehabilitation facility. He demonstrates a tremendous interest and passion for the field of speech and language pathology and works towards the best interests of his patients.

"I had the opportunity to speak with several patients and family members who interacted and worked with Mr. Ittleman and all were most complimentary about his treatment style and his emphasis on getting them back into conversation. Patients have conveyed to me that Mr. Ittleman understands what is most meaningful to patients who have lost the ability to communicate with their family and peers day in and day out. He works with them to get them back using both conversation and the technology that they were used to working with in their lives.

"It is for this reason that I would recommend Mr. Ittleman for any position in which he can serve the population he is passionate about. His direct patient care is an asset to the profession. " **S. Andrews**

Testimonials from New Speech Pathologists

"Mark, Thank you for making my transition into this Rehabilitation Agency so wonderful! I really appreciate all your support and time, especially to answer my randomly timed questions. You have made such a positive impact on the way I practice! Thank You!!" Sincerely, **E. Mathukutty**

"Dear Mark, Thank you so much for your overwhelming love and compassion to help me grow and succeed especially as a fresh fish in the pond. I am very honored to have moved you to write more in your book. You are an amazing teacher and I thank you in advance for having the heart, passion, and determination to share your skills with the world. We are still colleagues in this field, although I am like a premie at this point, and I look forward to working with you here and in other areas in the future. Thanks again, Mark, for making me feel like a person with a possible future in this field and not just any other student. Thanks again!" **C. Davis**

Testimonials from Speech Pathology Students

"Dear Mark, I just want to say thank you for being an inspiration in my path of becoming a speech-language pathologist. I truly enjoyed every moment I spent observing your interactions with patients and seeing your methods work wonders. As I continue along with my career endeavors, I hope to follow along in your footsteps. It brings me pleasure to know that through your techniques and new website, people anywhere in the world will have the opportunity to use a fun and proven way to help their loved ones speak again. Once again, thanks for being such a wonderful mentor." **N. Vera**, Undergraduate Student at University of Houston.

"During the summer of 2011, I had a wonderful life experience. I was able to observe Mark for a few days in his speech therapy sessions. They were very interesting because he was having actual conversations with people who could hardly talk!

The conversations were very interesting because they were with stroke patients and brain injured people. He was able to get them to communicate in conversation in a way they felt secure and understood. Mark made them feel that they mattered.

Mark invited me to come and observe his sessions since I was inquiring about becoming a speech-language pathologist. That experience opened my heart to what could be done in conversation. He had a structure to what he was doing, and was asking questions that were easy for the patients to answer. What was interesting was that the questions he asked them practically had the answers in them, and they were meaningful.

I was honored to hear about a patient's passion for music, the conversation of a mom talking about her teenager, and another person who talked about a trip taken to Las Vegas. It was also interesting to hear a father talk about his relationship with his son.

It was delightful and inspiring. Above all, it touched my heart and inspired me to become a speech pathologist!

Thank you Mark!!!"

M. Elizondo

the teaching TALKING

**Learn to Do Expert
Speech Therapy at Home**
—WITH CHILDREN AND ADULTS—

Mark A. Ittleman, M.S., CCC/SLP.

The speech pathologist who can make rocks talk!

New York

the teaching of TALKING
Learn to Do Expert Speech Therapy at Home
—WITH CHILDREN AND ADULTS—

ISBN 978-1-61448-253-6 paperback
ISBN 978-1-61448-254-3 eBook
Library of Congress Control Number: 2012933652

Morgan James Publishing
The Entrepreneurial Publisher
5 Penn Plaza, 23rd Floor,
New York City, New York 10001
(212) 655-5470 office • (516) 908-4496 fax
www.MorganJamesPublishing.com

Cover Design by:
Rachel Lopez
www.r2cdesign.com

Interior Design by:
Bonnie Bushman
bonnie@caboodlegraphics.com

In an effort to support local communities, raise awareness and funds, Morgan James Publishing donates a percentage of all book sales for the life of each book to Habitat for Humanity Peninsula and Greater Williamsburg.

Get involved today, visit
www.MorganJamesBuilds.com.

Note to the Reader

Welcome, Reader! You know, when Malka and I have friends over for the first time, we "show them around" so they can get a feel for our home. Likewise, I invite you to take a tour of this treatise on *The Teaching of Talking*. Come in. Take a look around. Then you'll know if what we have to share will be right and comfortable for you. We hope so.

You will find within these pages a unique method to help people speak. This book will show you how you can learn to provide expert speech therapy to help your clients or loved ones. It is designed for the speech pathologist, family members, and caregivers. Just about anyone can learn this method to help someone speak. I know, because in the last 40 years I have taught hundreds of people to help their loved ones speak again.

We would point you to the *Conclusion* on page 163, where you will find a summary of our beliefs. Our unique approach to the teaching of talking can be found in the chapters following *Stimulating Speech and Language* on page 43. After your stop at the *Conclusion*, we would direct you to the section entitled, *Who This Book Will Help*, on page 41. These pages provide some screening tests that will help you determine whether this text would be a good "fit" for your client, loved one, or patient.

The book you are holding contains the secrets to helping others speak. Reading it could be one of the most important things you ever do. You have the potential to alter and improve another person's life by learning and applying the methods contained in *The Teaching of Talking*.

Thank you so much for stopping by! Please visit our website, www.teachingoftalking.com. I hope you will use the methods in this book to become a *teacher of talking* for your clients or loved one!

I remain very truly yours,
Mark

Readers: We have prepared a survey that we would ask you to complete before you begin reading *The Teaching of Talking*, and a second survey that we would ask you to complete after you have finished it. Together, these surveys will provide valuable feedback regarding what you, our readers, have learned from this text, and whether you believe this knowledge will help as you work with your client or loved one. *These easy-to-use surveys can be completed online at our site, www. teachingoftalking.com.* Please remember not to take the "Post-Reading Survey" until you have completely read *The Teaching of Talking*! Thank you for helping us to serve you better! We will send you something of value in appreciation for completing both surveys.

Mark

Dedication

This book is dedicated to my wonderful wife, Malka.
You have enabled me to be the "King of my Castle"
and have allowed me the freedom
to devote my energies
to the pursuit of *The Teaching of Talking*
and the completion of this text.
You have also afforded me the opportunity
to use the principles
of *The Teaching of Talking*
to help you gain speaking
confidence and competence when
speaking the English language.

I love you dearly.

I would also like to dedicate this text to the late I.A. Weinstein, who helped guide me into the field of speech pathology; to Beth Valerie (Stein) Stone, a study partner, who helped me get through undergraduate work in speech pathology; and to Bonnie, my ex-wife, who worked alongside me throughout my twenty years of private practice in Lakeland, Florida.

Thank you to the late Dr. Charles Van Riper, whose textbooks I studied as a student. His writings helped to instill in me a love for the field I would soon pursue, and his words and clinical advice often resonate within me. Dr. Van Riper commented in his text: "We hope that a new generation of students, like those who have studied this text for almost forty years, will sense the challenge of trying to help those who cannot share our common heritage, the ability to communicate effectively."[1]

It is my hope that this text, *The Teaching of Talking, Learn to Do Expert Speech Therapy at Home with Children and Adults*, will pose a similar challenge to future generations of students. Like my esteemed colleague, Dr. Van Riper, I have served as a clinician my entire career and I have enjoyed every minute of it. I hope that enjoyment permeates these pages.

---

1   Charles VanRiper, Speech Correction, Principle and Methods , 6th ed.(Englewood Cliffs, NJ: Prentice-Hall, 1978), 1.

Contents

Preface

As a beginning speech-language pathologist, I had no clue what to do for people who were unable to talk. I had learned theoretical principles and approaches to speech and language therapy. Now, I thought, I just need to show my patients who cannot speak some picture cards, ask them what the pictures are, buy some training manuals for aphasia, copy the exercises, and have them fill in the blanks.

Wrong! It was not that easy for me, and I knew it. I was bewildered. I had some ideas about how I wanted to help people talk, and so far, I had no proof that the theories and principles I had been taught were working. There is nothing more frustrating than to be in a situation where someone is depending on you, and you don't have the answer, or to think you have the answer, and quickly learn that you do not.

Despite my frustration at not knowing what would really work for people who could not speak, I went about practicing the art of speech-language therapy in 1972, when I received the Certificate of Clinical Competence in Speech Language Pathology. I studied, attended seminars, and read everything I could on the subject; and somehow, through time, I got a grasp on what I believed to be the true fundamentals of success in helping both children and adults speak with clarity.

The fundamental principle I learned was to train family members or caregivers to do what I did in speech therapy and to assure myself that they were able to do it as well as I could. That way, they could go home and continue to stimulate language and carry over what had been started in the therapy office. My students became not only the individuals who had mild to profound speaking difficulties, but their family members and caregivers as well. In time, family members and caregivers learned what they needed to do in order to help their loved ones speak better. They were amazed at the progress their loved ones made with a team approach to speech therapy.

Speech-language pathology students at nearby colleges came and worked with me during their clinical fellowship year, and they went on to "pay it forward" with the people who would come to them for therapy.

It took me years to develop these methods. Now I wish to share them with speech-language pathologists, loved ones, and caregivers throughout the nation and the world. Speech-language pathology has been very good to me, and I have decided to devote the rest of my working life to making sure that others will not have to spend five, ten, twenty, thirty, or forty years of practice to finally "get it right."

Consumers — including speech-language pathologists, family members, and caregivers — have spent millions of dollars each and every year buying manuals, computer programs, and other methods that purport to help the stroke patient or child speak again. Unfortunately, many have been disappointed in the results of these products. It is unfortunate that consumers buy products they think will help, only to discover within the first few times they are used that they have limited or no benefit.

No machine or computer is capable of assessing the many approaches that may be necessary to help someone regain their ability to speak. The most important need an individual experiencing communication difficulty has in order to successfully learn or relearn speech is a person willing to serve as a speech model (SM). Having models to learn from is the only way to develop speech and language. The way to learn or relearn speech and language is to have SMs accessible who will speak and stimulate language.

No magic potion, pill, or "device" will be the answer to teaching your patient or loved one to talk. The resource that will work for your patient or loved one is a human being who cares enough to search ceaselessly for methods and techniques that will be appropriate and beneficial for them. This will be a therapist, teacher, friend, loved one, or caregiver.

The Teaching of Talking is about speech therapists, speech-language pathologists, caregivers, family members, and health care professionals learning successful ways to stimulate people to speak and use language. Our company, *Be in Conversation PLLC*, has taken a committed stand to help people communicate and speak, which is vital in the fulfillment of life potential. Our purpose is to train people to provide speech and language stimulation for those who do not speak or for those who have lost that ability. We offer books, audio recordings, live seminars, and webinars to bring this information to people throughout the country and the world who have the daunting responsibility or a strong desire to help people talk. We will also be available as a resource to those who may need special mentoring or coaching through live video conferencing on the World Wide Web.

Mark A. Ittleman, M.S., CCC/SLP
Speech-Language Pathologist
Houston, Texas
December 2011

Acknowledgments

The Teaching of Talking has been my brainchild since beginning Landmark Education four years ago. At this life-changing program, I learned something very important about the purpose of human life: *it is not all about me!* In fact, the opposite is true: life, when properly lived, is about making a contribution to humanity and making a difference. So I first thank my friends at Landmark Education.

Some years ago, I had the opportunity to work with four patients who had profound expressive aphasia of the Broca's-type. We were together five days a week, eight hours per day. I knew intuitively and professionally that speech and language should be stimulated in conversation within activities of daily living (ADLs), in single words, phrases, and sentences. To assist me with these patients, I trained a Certified Nursing Assistant (CNA) with a high school education and found that she could learn to stimulate speech and language with profoundly aphasic people as competently as any speech-language pathologist I had ever met.

I thank my colleagues, patients, and their families at The Institute for Research and Rehabilitation (TIRR) at Memorial Hermann Hospital — Kirby Glen, Houston, Texas, which is the finest outpatient rehabilitation center in the country. The patients and staff there have challenged my creativity and personal resources. I am also thankful to Kathy Carrico, MSW, who encouraged me to establish a teaching relationship with the *Stroke Warriors of Houston* in order to help the participants and family members understand crucial principles for the improvement of speaking. I am also thankful to the speech pathology team at TIRR and a host of others too numerous to mention.

I am especially indebted to Elizabeth Mathukutty, M.S., Speech-Language Pathologist at TIRR, for her support and collaborative efforts in this *The Teaching of Talking* endeavor. I would also like to thank Caitlind Davis, M.S., CFY, Clinical Fellow in Speech-Language Pathology.

To a very skillful team of editors, George and Barbara Skipworth, thank you for your contribution to this text.

And, finally, I would like to thank Brittney Heath, Executive Assistant, and Wendy Leonard, Editor, for our Company, *Be in Conversation PLLC*. They have helped me take this project to a national and international level. Their commitment and shared passion to take our message to the world has been an inspiration.

Introduction

The ability to speak and to be understood is an ability that many of us take for granted. We know that when we open our mouth, words will surface and be expressed. Words are essential in human relationships. We learn, interact, develop relationships, express love, and work through the use of words. What happens to the life of a child whose speech does not develop properly? What happens to people who lose the ability to speak because of a stroke or brain injury?

This book is about helping children and adults who have lost the ability to speak. It focuses on teaching you, the reader, how to use techniques I have spent forty years developing to help your loved one cultivate or regain the ability to speak. For the speech-language pathologist who is reading this book, it will help you become more effective in your approach to helping people talk.

If I could sum this book up in a few paragraphs, it would be this:

You will learn how to help people talk again. The method will be conversational in nature, in that you will help people recover the ability to speak as you *talk* to them using words at their level. You will learn how to step into their world, to speak with them about what really lights them up, and to show them how to expand what they are saying from single words to two-word combinations, then to phrases, and eventually to complete sentences. What is best about this method is the lack of "homework." Your *therapy* consists of encouraging them to talk all through the day in whatever activities you do together. What could be more enjoyable than that?

This book was written with the family member, caregiver, or speech-language pathologist in mind. It does not include a lot of theory. You will be stimulating talking at home, where speech is first learned; and the person who will be modeling correct speech will be the one who loves or cares for the person who has difficulty speaking. Do you see the simplicity in that?

Why do I not include a lot of theory? Most books about speech improvement are just that, a lot of theory with no meat, no method, no systematic technique, or structure. I went to college for years and was hard pressed to find one book that taught me how to teach someone to talk.

One of my mentors, Ace Weinstein, once said that it doesn't matter what college you go to....they all have the same textbooks. He also said that college is all theory, and life after graduation is all practice. This book is about teaching someone to talk or talk again, and you will begin practicing as you read. Start right away! Don't wait. Jump right in and read as you go along. Help your loved one or client speak again.

As long as the person you are working with fits the criteria for this method (see pages 23-28), you should see results! Speech recovery may be very slow or may be rapid. Either way, the race for speech recovery will begin with you.

A word of warning: This book is not intended to replace the services of a speech-language pathologist, but to supplement the work you will be doing with one. Later, after discharge, it can be used to help you move to more complex levels of language stimulation. You must be dedicated and realize there are no quick fixes. The most valuable things we obtain in life are gained through blood, sweat, and tears.

I love you, dear reader, and know you are embracing a task that may at first seem insurmountable. The fruits of your labor will come with faith and determination. I challenge you not to take this venture on lightheartedly. It may consume you as it has me, and I have loved every minute of the ride. With this book, my bus is stopping for you to get on. Stimulating speech and language is a way of life. Come with me and let me show you what is possible!

Mark A. Ittleman, M.S., CCC/SLP
"The speech pathologist who can make rocks talk!"
December, 2011
Houston, Texas

The Teaching of Talking — A Conversational Approach to Helping the Person with a Mild to Profound Speech and Language Impairment Talk Better

The *Teaching of Talking* is a new approach to speech and language therapy. It is a very different method in comparison to the traditional way in which aphasic patients are being treated today. Dr. Joseph Wepman, who treated soldiers returning home from war with traumatic brain injuries and aphasia in the 1950s, initially established the traditional school of thought about speech and language therapy for stroke patients or those with head injuries. In 1980, Dr. Frederic Darley, Mayo Clinic, Rochester, New York; Dr. Nancy A Helm, Veterans Administration Medical Center, Boston, Massachusetts; Dr. Audrey Holland, University of Pittsburgh, Pennsylvania; and Craig Linebaugh, George Washington University, Washington, D.C., [1] led a panel discussion regarding techniques for treating mild or high-level aphasic impairments. Darley, et al. (1980) commented on the change of heart Dr. Joseph Wepman expressed concerning the speech and language stimulation approach for individuals with aphasia. (Darley, June 1-5, 1980)

---

1   Frederic L. Darley, et al., "Techniques in Treating Mild or High-level Aphasic Impairment" (Proceedings of the 10th Clinical Aphasiology Conference, June 1-5, 1980), Clinical Aphasiology Conference (Bar Harbor, ME: BRK Publishers, 1980): 338-345, accessed March 2011, http://aphasiology.pitt.edu/archive/00000565/.

(Wepman 1951) "Joseph Wepman in his 1951 book, Recovery from Aphasia, described as a useful regimen the teaching first of a series of nouns, then at a given level of adequacy of retrieval of those nouns, the teaching of verbs to go with them. So one might teach the nouns "knife" and "chair," then the verbs "cut" and "sit," and then go on to sentences such as "The knife cuts." Twenty-five years later, Wepman has come to advise something quite different. He downgrades work on language as language. He believes that concentration on words leads to a struggle for accuracy in word finding that interferes with thought. He reminds us that it should be the other way around —that thought should be stimulated, which in turn leads to words as a means of its expression. He points out that speech should be the handmaiden of thought, not its master and controller. He advises us to stimulate the patient to think and allow to occur whatever verbal behavior the patient is capable of producing. We should keep the flow of ideas going, directing it toward the specific area of thought one has selected. He likens this process to what Weigl described as deblocking: reorganize the higher mental processes and permit the lower levels (that is, language comprehension and its use) to emerge."

I strongly concur with Wepman and also believe that individuals with a severe to profound speech and language loss must first be "primed," like the old-fashioned water pump.[2] We must first prepare the person who is not speaking through very simple language stimulation methods that *require thought* and structuring simple language utterances during *activities of daily living (ADL)*, such as those developed in *The Teaching of Talking*. Speech is stimulated by first asking a question, which requires *thought* by the person it is directed toward, prior to their answer. Once the individual is able to *think* and answer the question with simple spoken language, speaking *confidence* improves. The focus of therapy continues to be stimulating *thought* with simple to more advanced questions, which in turn leads to increased expansion and expression of spoken words. Wepman had a change of heart about the approach to aphasia therapy after twenty-five years of practice, but I don't want you or the people you serve to have to wait that long.

This text and the procedures contained herein are the result of over forty years of experience providing speech and language stimulation to individuals

2   "Priming the pump: a procedure of introducing fluid into a pump to get the water flowing," in The Free Dictionary, s.v., "pump+priming," accessed July 2011, http://thefreedictionary.com/pump+priming.

who either did not develop speech and language normally due to developmental problems, hearing loss, or mental retardation; or those who acquired speech and language loss following a life-threatening incident such as a motor vehicle accident, head injury, stroke, or neurological insult. There is a wide diversity of age and cause among those people who suffer from speech and language difficulties.

Language is a shared system for communicating and exchanging knowledge, feelings, thoughts, and beliefs. It involves sounds, signs, gestures, and spoken or written words that convey meanings within a group or community.[3] When this normal process is interrupted or disabled, it may considerably affect the individual's ability to learn and communicate with others, which in turn can have a profound impact on social and business relationships, job performance, and earning capability.

The purpose of this book is to encourage the speech-language pathologist to look at the stimulation of speech and language in a way that is quite natural, involving current life routines and events of daily living. It is also written for parents, spouses, loved ones, and caregivers of those with speech and language difficulties, in the hope that they can provide speech and language stimulation at home, which is where most speech and language is initially developed.

The "Grandfather of Speech Therapy," Dr. Charles Van Riper stated, "Libraries are crammed with books on how to teach everything from advertising to zoology, but you will search long and far for a book on the teaching of talking, the most useful of all our communicative skills."[4] Although times have changed in the last fifty years, there is still an incredible need for *user friendly* books and digital, audio/video information that is simple enough for anyone to learn the methods for helping people talk.

Individuals with whom I have worked through the years have made significant improvement in the ability to speak and communicate with the assistance of loving parents, spouses, or caregivers who have learned the methods provided within the speech therapy environment and then went on to apply those same methods at home. Some of the best stimulators of language I have found are loving support personnel who do everything possible to help the person speak. Whether you are a speech-language pathologist, public health nurse, parent,

---

3   "Speech and Language Developmental Milestones," National Institute on Deafness and Other Communication Disorders, National Institutes of Health , Bethesda, MD 20892-2320, June, 2010, http://www.nidcd.nih.gov/health/voice/pages/speechandlanguage.aspx.

4   Charles Van Riper, Speech Correction, Principles and Methods, 3rd ed. (Englewood Cliffs, NJ: Prentice –Hall, 1954), 93.

spouse or caregiver, you can make a valuable contribution to helping others talk and communicate. Therefore, this book has been written with you in mind.

Who Are the People Who Need Us?

The people who need us are those who do not speak at all or those who have a great deal of difficulty speaking. They did not learn to talk during the language formulation years, or they had the ability to speak but lost it due to a neurological disease or trauma. The people who need us are often shy, lonely, and out of communication with those they love. Many prefer *not* to speak due to their disability and may withdraw into what I call the "closet of life." They may refuse to answer the phone, go to church, and participate in family events. Adults who lose the ability to speak with clarity may refuse to see friends and decline social opportunities. They isolate themselves and prefer to be "locked away" in their closet of life.

Children who do not develop speech normally find themselves rejected and ridiculed by their normal-speaking peers. Due to their difficulty with self-expression and frustration at not being understood, they may act out and develop behavioral problems, seeking the attention of others in negative ways as a result of their limited verbal expression. Academic achievement is often compromised, since the child may arrive at school for the first time without having mastered the sounds of speech, and yet facing the almost impossible task of learning how to read and write. That would be like leaving on a ten mile hike with no shoes or socks and wearing nothing but a pair of *Fruit of the Looms*!

The Speech Model

To improve speech and language for the child or adult, we must have a speech model (SM), since the person with the communication difficulty (PCD) must be able to hear what is said and then repeat the words spoken. Since human beings first develop speech by being exposed to SMs — mothers, fathers, caregivers, friends, teachers, etc. — we can surmise that the same principles would apply to those who have lost their ability to speak.

There are products that include computer programs, textbooks, and other media; but it is my sincere belief that there is no better way for a person to improve speech than with a good speaking model who is lively and interactive in nature, such as another human being *in the moment*. Therefore, before we start, a good SM is a prerequisite for the individual with a mild to profound speaking difficulty. A certified speech-language pathologist familiar with

The Teaching of Talking methodology should evaluate the PCD's speaking and language difficulties and inform you whether the PCD is stimulable for speech therapy.

Motor Speech Disorders

Before embarking on a project of helping another to speak well, you must have an understanding of what the individual can and cannot do in terms of their speaking ability. This is also necessary to establish a prognosis for future potential. The evaluation of speech by a certified speech-language pathologist will often include the status of an individual's articulation, or the ability to produce the sounds of one's native language.

Sadly, not everyone is capable of speaking, even with the best of teachers. Therefore, we will be addressing the speech and language needs of people who are capable of producing the vowels: (a, e, i, o, u), single syllable words (bus, car, one, eye, hand, food, etc.) or word pairs (more milk, go out, go sleep, read book, etc.). If the person is capable of saying the vowels after you, or if they can repeat simple single words with the model you give them, then we have potential and possibility for improvement of speaking using speech and language stimulation techniques. *Stimulation* is to encourage and excite a new speaking behavior that will replace the unwanted or absent speech-related behavior.

There are those who are unable to repeat vowels, single syllables, or word pairs after you. *Imitation* involves sitting directly across from someone and asking them to repeat after you. Some people with severe speech and language difficulties also have *apraxia of speech*, which is an inability to voluntarily imitate vowels, speech sounds, words, or word combinations. In the case of a severe to profound apraxia of speech, the individual may have significant difficulty getting the speech "motor" to perform the task of articulating and enunciating the sounds contained within the spoken word. If a PCD cannot imitate even the simplest of vowel sounds, they will not be a good candidate for *The Teaching of Talking* methods. If so, a method to address apraxia of speech is recommended. We plan to address this technique in a future publication.

A *peripheral oral examination* is also included in the assessment of speech and language by a speech-language pathologist. This examination tests the structures of the speech mechanism, which include the lips, teeth, tongue, palate, and soft palate to see if they are functioning adequately for the production of speech. The motor speech mechanism includes these structures which are put into motion by nerves and muscles to produce articulate speech and language.

Articulation is the formation of sounds with the structures of the mouth. The lips are responsible for the articulation of (p), (b), (m), (w), (f), and (v); and the teeth are responsible for the articulation of (f), (v), and voiced-voiceless (th). The tongue is responsible for the articulation of (t), (d), (n), (l), (sh), (ch), and (g), as in "beige," as well as the "hard" (k) and (g). One must have the potential to articulate accurately in order to be understood by others.

Speech intelligibility is a determination expressed by the speech pathologist in a percentage (the higher the percentage, the higher the speech intelligibility) that deals with whether speech is readily understood by the listener. It is dependent upon how well the motor speech mechanism is operating to make accurate speech sounds and how readily others understand what is being said.

> **Example**: If an individual has 50% speech intelligibility, half of what is said is understood; 75%, three quarters of what is said is understood.

Intelligibility may be influenced by the articulation, speed, or manner of speaking. Speech intelligibility judgments may also vary depending on factors related to the listener and whether they are familiar with the speaker.

Dysarthria of Speech

One factor that is affected in people with stroke or brain injury is the speed at which they do things. They often walk, talk, think, and perform tasks more slowly than those who are not brain-injured. Often, in the case of an acquired deficit, an individual may have been speaking at a particular speed for many years. If there is dysarthria, or slurred speech, the person with a communication difficulty (PCD) may be attempting to speak at their *habitual speed*. This is the speed at which they have always spoken. When someone speaks at their habitual speed with a less-than-intact motor speech system, the result will be slurred speech. It is often difficult to decipher what people are saying, since the speech sounds are not made accurately and therefore distort and are unclear.

Stroke and neurological trauma can affect motor skills, which often slow down the performance of walking, swallowing, reading, writing, math, and speech. In the case of speech, the motor may no longer be able to articulate the sounds within the words at its accustomed habitual speed. Therefore, if the PCD attempts to speak at the habitual speed, the resulting speech will be severely slurred. The lips, tongue, and palate cannot move at the speed they once did. Therefore, the individual with a speaking difficulty must learn to adjust the speed for more accurate speech. Although speech may be very slurred or distorted, it is difficult to change one's normal speech rate due to years of habitually speaking that way.-

Even though their speech may be difficult for others to decipher, PCDs often cannot immediately adjust their speaking rate and *latency* (the separation between words) independently. We often speak without consciously thinking because everything about speaking, for those with or without an acquired deficit, is automatic. Those with acquired speech deficits find themselves slurring speech and cannot seem to change that practice because their speaking rate became an established habit prior to having acquired a speech difficulty. Our *Make Every Word Count©* Seminar, which will be available in the near future, deals with dysarthria (the slurring of speaking) and will teach the caregiver and speech-language pathologist how to help those with slurred speech talk with clarity.

Our job as a speech model is to demonstrate an optimum speed of talking that will help the PCD coordinate the rate of their thinking with slower speech. Slowing down to an optimum speaking speed will allow them more time to formulate what they want to say and the speed at which they wish to say it. Often, when the speed of speaking is slowed down and the PCD is shown how to pause between each word spoken, the tongue, lips, and palate will work with improved accuracy, resulting in more intelligible speech. Therapy to address optimum speaking speed, latency, or language usage is like developing any "new habit." New habits must be repeated until they finally become subconscious, much like the learning of the alphabet, times tables, layout of a new workplace, or navigation of city streets. Learning a foreign language is a similar process; one must repeat the new words and phrases often and slowly before it becomes "automatic."

Defining and Testing of Receptive and Expressive Language

Receptive language is the ability to understand what is spoken or written. During a typical speech evaluation, the speech-language pathologist will test an individual with a speaking difficulty using standardized and informal testing measurements. Standardized tests compare the individual with others of a similar age or speech difficulty, and informal testing documents what the individual is actually doing when they communicate.

Standardized tests are often developed in a university setting using hundreds of participants. At the conclusion of testing, the speech-language pathologist is able to compute a score based on the performance of the individual. Each score is compared to the group of participants initially tested. Standardized tests often have pictures and require the individual to point to the "correct one," or the person may be instructed to follow simple or complex directions. These tests measure how well one recognizes and comprehends spoken and written language.

Expressive language is the ability to speak and use written language to express oneself. The expressive language portion of the standardized assessment documents a person's ability to produce words and construct phrases or sentences while speaking or writing. It also includes the ways in which individuals use nouns, verbs, tenses, phrases, sentences, and simple grammar.

Informal testing is an observation of social interaction and communication between two or more people. We are watching and listening for the sounds of speech, voice quality and loudness, the rate of speech, word usage, vocabulary, comprehension, mannerisms, and attending behaviors.

Language Samples

Language samples are the tools that speech-language pathologists (SLP) use to document what is spoken. The SLP records the grammar, syntax, or word order of the individual's speech. This requires *transcription,* or the ability to write down everything an individual says. This is subsequently analyzed to determine how well one uses the "rules" of the language. Language sample analysis tools may vary from a pen and a legal pad to newer ways of analysis through the use of computer technology, speech recognition software, and language sample analysis software (Parrot Software, SALT Software, etc.).

Many choose to complete an informal language sample because of the versatility of this tool; that is, it allows the professional to examine as much or as little linguistic information as is necessary to fill in the gaps from the formal assessment profile. The standardized assessment tools are only a starting point and should be used in conjunction with observations and informal assessments. SLPs should be skilled in the assessment of speech and language functioning and use both informal and formal assessments to get a better overview of the individual's communication abilities.[5]

---

5   "Speech Language Assessment; Target: Texas Guide for Effective Teaching," (Speech Language Assessment; Texas Statewide Leadership for Autism Training, March 2009), 7.

Following are excerpts of two early language samples taken from my therapy sessions with Ray.[6] Language samples taken at the conclusion of therapy are on page 135 of this text.

I tut rat and wee eetid. (I cut grass and weed eated.)
A tee sop (at the shop)
She hant haw afor me. (She can't afford me.)
No.
I don't want to tut tas. (I don't want to cut grass.)
I soo. (I do.)
She mase me sim and all. (She makes me??)
Is on huh (??)

I ----- senk 4 uh uh coffee. (I drink 4 cups of coffee.)
No.
I work (I worked)
I wort at sepis taytin (I worked at a service station)
Huf (Gulf)
I humph hass (I pumped gas)
I wat tisteen (I was sixteen)
Tah der (dollar)
I was matin a dah der (I was makin a dollar)
I was wortin to mate a buck (??)
I wuh nun no (I wouldn't know)

From the language sample, we are able to identify possible breakdowns in talking. Next, we can formulate a plan to address one or more of the following areas: voice, articulation, speed, pacing of speech, and the expression of thought into words. There are PCDs who may also be given tests of *stimulability*. This involves identifying the problematic speaking habit and providing a simple, accurate model of the desired speech behavior. If the PCD can accurately duplicate the good model of speech provided by the SM, then their stimulability is good. If the PCD is unable to accurately duplicate the SM, it typically means

---

6   Names have been changed throughout this manuscript to protect the privacy of patients.

that the task we have given them is too difficult, and we need to find a simpler way to present it or find some other speech behavior to stimulate.

Tests of stimulability are also used by the speech-language pathologist to determine where to begin improving speech; i.e., vowel, consonant, syllable, single word, phrase, sentence level, voice, pitch, loudness, or speed in speaking. Therefore, if I find something about someone's speech that could use improvement, I model how it should be correctly produced, and ask the PCD to repeat that model after me. If they can produce the new model with instruction, their stimulability will be good for that task. Prognosis for improvement is often a reflection of the PCD's stimulability.

The Importance of Vocabulary

Vocabulary is a reflection of who you are. It is part of the foundation for speaking and determines how well you are able to share your thoughts with others. This program, *The Teaching of Talking*, is about using simple words to share your thoughts with others and to make simple requests.

Alla Zareva, Ph.D. (2008), in an article about vocabulary size of *native speakers* (NS), defined a native speaker's language as learned from birth or as the language that a multi-lingual person speaks the best. Zareva reported that native speakers have a highly organized vocabulary of several thousand words, with conservative estimates at 14,000 to 20,000 words. She furthermore states that more liberal studies suggest 50,000 words and more. These studies also report that native speakers can access these words very quickly (200 milliseconds) upon recognition. Zareva states that native speakers are surprisingly fast at finding words they need when speaking. Native Speakers (NS) maintain a speaking rate (speed) of about 150 words per minute, which computes to a recall speed of about one-third of a second to retrieve a word desired for a simple phrase or sentence.[7]

Those of us who speak with PCDs realize it may take several seconds for some to achieve *name recall*[8] of a word or a thought that is difficult to express, and they may also have *verbal paraphasic*[9] *errors,* which occur when the word which is

---

7   Alla Zareva, Ph.D., "Frontier Words in the L2 Mental Lexicon," Ohio University Working Papers in Linguistics and Language Teaching (2008), accessed on March 2011, http://www.ohiou.edu/linguistics/workingpapers/2008/zareva_2008.pdf.

8   Sandy A. Starch and Robert C. Marshall, "Who's on First? A Treatment Approach for Name Recall with Aphasic Patients." (16th In Clinical Aphasiology Conference, June 8-12, 1986), Clinical Aphasiology Conference (Jackson, WY: BRK Publishers, 1986).

9   Patrick McCaffrey, Ph.D., " CMSD 636 Neuro-Pathologies of Language and Cognition, Chapter 5. Aphasia-Concomitant Characteristics," The Neurosciences on the Web Series, 2011, accessed on

desired for recall is substituted by another word which was not intended. *Anomia* occurs with aphasia, dementia, and cognitive difficulties, and is also associated with word-finding difficulties, and occurs when one attempts to recall the name of an acquaintance or a specific word. *Circumlocutions* (speaking in a roundabout way) occur when the PCD cannot recall the word attempted and other related or nonrelated words are expressed instead. Often, the word can be recalled when partially started or repeated after the SM.

Imagine for a moment what it would be like if you did not have a word for places you wanted to go, for the things you needed, the emotions you felt on a daily basis, or dreams you would like to accomplish or share with others. It would be a world in which your mind would be devoid of pictures or thoughts. Or, it would be like seeing or hearing the word you want to say in your mind, but being unable to say it. One of the best ways I could describe this is when you see someone you know, and your memory of their name is temporarily unavailable. Have you ever found yourself in a situation where you could not find your keys, and you realized they were in the car, but the car was locked? All you could do was look in through the car window, *see* the keys inside the car, say a few expletives, and realize you could not get in the car because all the windows were closed and the doors were locked! You could *see* the keys, but you had *no access* into the car.

People with moderate to profound speaking difficulties may be able to see or hear the word in their minds, but they are unable to transmit the word or thought to the lips, teeth, and tongue. If you think about the words you have to generate when speaking, they would be subdivided into categories. All of the words that one understands and expresses are called the lexicon or vocabulary. Think about all the words you or the PCD think about each day. These words can be classified according to some of the following categories.

Throughout this book you will see small scroll icons. The scroll brings your attention to words you should record on a computer, in a notebook, or on an iPad or other digital device for use with your PCD. This will help you become more aware of vocabulary that you will be stimulating.
All lists referred to in The Teaching of Talking are available in Word format at www.teachingoftalking.com.

January 2012, http://www.csuchico.edu/~pmccaffrey/syllabi/SPPA336/336unit5.html.

Category	Words
Resting	bed, well, couch, chair, recliner, nap, sleep, bedroom
Feelings	well, not well, good, happy, sleepy, tired, aware
Toileting	now, pee, bowel movement (BM), poop
Bathing	bath, shower, water, shampoo, soap, towel, dry
Washing	warm, hot, soap, washcloth, face, hands, scrub
Grooming	brush, comb, gel, haircut, razor, shave
Dressing	clothing item, number of items, color, size, order of dressing
Eating	more, drink, hungry, juice, cereal, eggs, toast, hamburger, soup
Time of day	morning, afternoon, day, evening, night
Locations	neighborhood, city, state, country, continent, world
Numbers	1 to infinity
Body parts	arms, legs, finger, head, chest, stomach, back
Places	home, work, shopping, doctor, restaurant, museum
Names of people	husband, wife, children, mother, father, siblings
Using the telephone	hello, goodbye, call back, hold, can't talk, how are you?
Managing medications	take pills, no swallow, too big, pill lost, don't want
Maintaining the home	wash, sweep, dust, make bed, empty trash, clean
Managing finances	cash, check, money, bill, pay, late
Shopping and money	Wal-mart, Kroger, Food, Mall, Publix
Using transportation	Car, taxi, bus, Metro, train, subway, limo, van, motorcycle

Review

Who Are the People Who Need Us? The people who need us include those who do not speak at all or those who experience great difficulty speaking due to early developmental delays, brain injury, or neurological insult, or stroke. You may recognize them when they withdraw from social opportunities and isolate themselves into a *closet of life*. Children often suffer ridicule from their peers due to their limited verbal abilities, causing them to become behavior problems.

The Speech Model. A speech model is anyone willing to volunteer their time to work with and model speech for someone who needs them.

Motor Speech Disorders. Problems with the structure of the motor speech structure (lips, teeth, tongue, palate, muscles and nerves) can lead to problems producing vowels, single syllables, word pairs, articulation, and imitation.

Dysarthria of Speech. Compromised motor skills lead to slurred speech, slowness of speech and other activities, and difficulty articulating sounds. Dysarthria can sometimes be corrected by demonstrating the use of optimum speed when talking.

Defining and Testing of Receptive and Expressive Language. Receptive language involves the spoken and written words. Expressive language involves the ability to speak or write to express yourself. Problems speaking could be a result of either difficulty receiving the communication or in sending it back out. It is the SLP's responsibility to determine which problem may be causing speaking difficulties.

Language Samples. Language samples include the tools used by SLP's to evaluate how well one uses the "rules" of language. These samples identify breakdowns in talking, which help determine where to begin improving speech.

The Importance of Vocabulary. Our use of vocabulary reflects who you are. It is the very foundation of our speech and what we share with others.

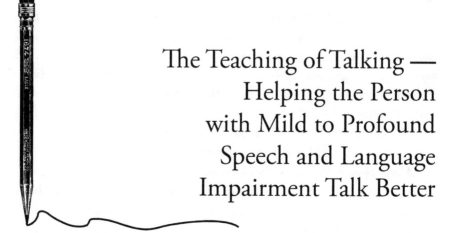

The Teaching of Talking —
Helping the Person
with Mild to Profound
Speech and Language
Impairment Talk Better

Speech and language stimulation should be like dancing with a good partner, smooth and fluid. The therapist or SM should be comfortable interacting with the PCD.

I am a speech and language model, and so are you. If you remember and utilize the fundamentals contained in this book, speaking will become easier and receptive and expressive language will improve for the PCD as a result of talking with you. If the PCD appears frustrated, it may be because the tasks you have given them are too difficult. However, you will soon learn what to do in order to make the whole process easier.

Why We Speak

If you look at your daily verbal interactions, they will be centered on an inquiry (the act of asking) and a reply (answering). The *inquiry is typically a question*: "Are you ready for breakfast?" "Did the mail come?" or "Would you like to see a movie?" An inquiry is also a request. A request *does not always have to be a question*. "I would like eggs this morning" or "I would like to write after breakfast." The last two statements could also be made into a question: "May I have eggs?" or "May I write after breakfast?" Either way, they represent what a person intends to do or desires from another person. Most communication is centered on inquiries, intentions, and general statements that express or reveal our thoughts. A general statement that may be a response to the question, "May I have eggs?" might be, "We are out of eggs. I will get some today."

Who Will This Book Help?

 This text is written to address the needs of persons with mild to profound speaking difficulties. A brief description of a person who would benefit from the strategies contained within this book is as follows:

Who will this book help?				
1	Is the PCD able to *follow simple directions?* Please check (√) "yes" or "no" if they can complete the following tasks at your request.			
		Yes	No	
	Please open your mouth			
	Please close your eyes			
	Please raise your hand			
	Please nod your head			
	Please shake your head			
	Please point up!			
	Please point down!			
	Please look down			
	Please look into my eyes			
	Please touch your ear			

Who will this book help?				
2	If the PCD can follow at least five of the requests above, they can follow a simple direction, and this is a positive prognostic factor. If they have difficulty, you can simplify the task to fewer words, as in the two-word requests below. Please check (√) "yes" or "no" if they can follow the *two-word directions* below.			
		Yes	**No**		
	Look up				
	Look down				
	Open mouth				
	Close mouth				
	Look right				
	Look left				
	Close eyes				
	Pucker lips				
	Smile				
	Nod head				
3	Is the PCD able to *articulate* the vowels accurately in imitation tasks? Please check (√) the "yes" or "no" column to indicate whether the PCD can repeat the following sounds after you:			
		Yes	**No**		
A	ah				
	ay				
	ae: (as in at)				
	ih: (as in it)				
	ai: (as in I)				
	oh				
	u (as in shoot)				

	Who will this book help?				
4	Is the PCD able to *imitate single syllable words* with reasonable accuracy, especially words which include the speech sounds: (p), (b), (m), and (w) with increasing complexity to the (t), (d), (n), (l), (s), (sh), (ch), (k), and (g)? Have the PCD repeat the words below after you, and check (√) whether you can or cannot understand the *initial speech sound* of each of the following words clearly.				
				Understood	Not Understood
	p:	pee			
	b:	bay			
	t:	tea			
	d:	day			
	n:	nay			
	l:	lay			
	s:	say			
	h:	hay			
	sh:	shy			
	ch:	chain			
	j:	John			
	k:	cool			
	f:	fair			
	v:	vain			
	th:	they			

Who will this book help?

5 | A *blend* is a combination of two consonant sounds before a vowel. They are usually harder to articulate if the child/adult is having difficulty with the production of speech sounds, whether it is developmental in nature or an acquired medical problem such as stroke, head injury, or neurological disease.

Is the PCD able to say the words below that start with initial blends, either repeating them after you or reading them from written copy? Please note: (1) is the ***blend*** articulated clearly and correctly, and (2) is the ***entire word*** pronounced so that you can understand it?

Check (√) "yes" or "no" *if the **blend** is articulated correctly*. If the ***entire word*** is clearly understood when it is repeated after you, check (√) "Understood." If you could not understand the entire word, then check (√) "Not Understood."

		Yes	No	Understood	Not Understood
bl:	blame				
cl:	clean				
fl:	flag				
gl:	glow				
pl:	play				
sl:	slow				
sk:	skate				
sw:	swim				
scr:	scrape				
str:	street				
spr:	spring				
sl:	slow				
sm:	smoke				
sn:	snow				
sp:	spoke				
st:	stove				
spl:	splatter				

Who will this book help?					
6	Is the PCD able to recite the following requests, independently or after you? They would be good candidates for *The Teaching of Talking* if they can do either task independently, or by repeating them after you. Please check the appropriate box.				
				Independent	Imitated
	Ask PCD to count from 1-10 (if they cannot do this independently, ask them to repeat after you)				
	Ask PCD to state the alphabet (if they cannot do this independently, ask them to repeat after you)				
	Ask PCD to name the days of the week (if they cannot do this independently, ask them to repeat after you)				
	Ask PCD to name the months of the year (if they cannot do this independently, ask them to repeat after you)				

Who will this book help?			
7	Is the PCD able to imitate one or two simple words together with intelligibility of at least 75% to 80%? Say the two-word phrases below, and have the PCD repeat the combinations after you. If they can repeat the two words, check the "two-word" column. If they have difficulty imitating two-word phrases, then have them repeat the same examples one word at a time; i.e., you would say "Love" and they would say "Love." Then say "You" and have them repeat "You." Put a check if they can say each word separately after you say each word. Please check (√) "two-word" if the PCD could say the two words as a phrase after you say the two words. If they could not repeat the two-word phrase, but they could repeat each individual word after you in the phrase, then check (√) "single-word." If they were unable to repeat the words in either task, check (√) "neither."		

	Two-word	Single-word	Neither
Love you.			
Miss you.			
Go now.			
Come here.			
Bye-bye			
Hello!			
Good night.			
Good day.			
I'm hungry.			
Water, please.			

Who will this book help?

8 | The PCD will demonstrate immediate memory and recall for what has been spoken and repeated with the speech-language pathologist, family, or caregivers. For example, if I show you how to say something, and you say it correctly and I ask you a few moments later (30 seconds) to say it again correctly, in this instance, the speech-language pathologist, family, or caregiver is looking to see whether the PCD can remember something that was previously stimulated.

An example of this would be the following:

"I am going to ask you to say the word '_____' in a moment or two." (Choose a specific word or phrase that the PCD has always used; such as office, coke, hamburger, TV, nap, eggs, beer, martini, bed, etc.) "I want you to remember this word because I will be asking you to repeat it again later in our conversation."

Or you could present the PCD with a concept or words that may be significant to the person. For example:

SM: "I know Elvis was one of your favorite singers, right? Say 'Elvis' right now."
PCD: "Elvis."
SM: "I will ask you in a few moments who one of your favorite singers was, and I want you to answer 'Elvis.' Okay?"

Continue talking with the PCD while you keep an eye on the clock. In about 30 seconds, interrupt your current discussion and ask the PCD, "Do you remember the word (or your favorite singer) that we talked about earlier? Can you repeat that word (name) now?"

Who will this book help?		
Check (√) the "30-second" box if the PCD is able to recall the word or name at the 30-second interval. Then continue your conversation, watching the clock for another 30 seconds. At the 60-second mark, again interrupt your conversation to see if the PCD can repeat the word or name they were supposed to remember. Check (√) the "60-second" box if the PCD is still able to recall the word or name at the 60-second interval.		
If they can recall the word or their favorite singer correctly, they have some immediate or recent recall. If they cannot, *that is okay*. You will start by asking questions using single words at the start of your speech and language work, and then progress to word pairs, phrases, and sentences. Immediate or recent recall often improves with practice.		
Stimulus Word (Make note of the stimulus word or question you choose)	30-second	60-second

If the PCD is not able to produce speech that you can understand, or if they are not able to perform the recall tasks, they may not be ready to pursue the fundamental procedures of *The Teaching of Talking* method of speech therapy.

You may nonetheless be considering some difficult persons for this approach. The major point I would like to make in spite of all the information I have given you is this:

As a speech-language pathologist, family member or caregiver, the two most important distinctions are (1) whether YOU and the person you are working with are dedicated to improving their speech, and (2) is the PCD stimulable? Can they imitate a vowel or even a simple single syllable word? (yes, no, bye, more, etc.) If they can, proceed with the procedures of *The Teaching of Talking*.

The Teaching of Talking is an appropriate approach for people who are able to accomplish any of the above tasks. If not, the PCD may have to undergo a different speech therapy approach before *The Teaching of Talking* is utilized. The people I see who are not ready for this approach are those who cannot follow simple directions or imitate the sounds of speech. Even with intensive models, they are not able to say vowels, or simple words of two to three consonants, such as (yes, no, ball, bed, car, pee, nap, or TV).

The Teaching of Talking was developed by a speech-language pathologist to be used with persons who have mild to profound speech and language difficulties. It is best used in coordination with a speech-language pathologist who is familiar with *The Teaching of Talking* methods. Our method (*The Teaching of Talking*) may also be used once the PCD has been discharged from active speech therapy as a home program to help them progress to more complex language utterances. At home, they can progress comfortably, since there are no time constraints or speech therapy limitations such as those set by insurance companies, speech therapy offices and outpatient clinics. The *Teaching of Talking* has structure that can be followed as the PCD recovers speech, therefore reducing the stress of having to get it done before the insurance or visits "run out."

Best efforts have been used to prepare the material presented. The author and publisher, however, cannot guarantee results with any of the methods contained within this text. Results in speech therapy vary greatly due to the background, experience, resources, ambitions, and individual effort put in by the PCDs themselves, as well as the "team" working with them. If great time and effort are not put into the teaching and practice of speaking all through the day, seven days a week, you may not attain the same results as another person would. Therefore, the author and publisher may not be held liable, in any circumstance, for damages or loss, including but not limited to special or incidental cases.

Review

Why we speak. We speak to answer inquiries and communicate with others.

Who will this book help? This book will help people with mild to profound speaking difficulties (1) if you are both committed to improving the PCD's speech and (2) if the PCD is stimulable.

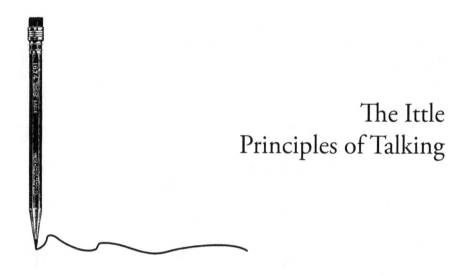

The Ittle
Principles of Talking

The First Ittle Principle —
Simplicity: Making It Easy

The first fundamental principle assures that what you are going to say to the individual will be easily grasped and repeated. *Always stimulate a person with words they can say after you with minimal effort*; that is, words that are very common, short or easy to say, often those having one syllable. Remember to say those words slowly and loudly enough, so that even a person with a hearing loss will catch it. If you do that, the PCD will gain confidence and respect for you and for the whole process of speech therapy. If the task is too difficult, they may use self-blame, self-criticism, or give up on the idea because speech and language stimulation (therapy) may be "too hard or frustrating."

The Second Ittle Principle — Speaking Clarity

If you are the individual who will be stimulating speech, we will refer to you and others like you as the speech model (SM): The individual or therapist who models correct articulation, pronunciation, grammar, sentence structure, and repetition of single words, phrases, or sentences, to help build correct speech and language skills in the PCD (person with communication difficulties). As the SM, you must have accurate speech, diction, loudness and speaking clarity to be heard and understood. If not, you are set up for failure, and it is probably best not to even start stimulation. If you are the SM, it is imperative that you speak loud enough to make an impression on the person with whom you are communicating. The PCD must be able to hear every sound, syllable, word, phrase, or sentence clearly so that they can accurately imitate what you have just said. The PCD should like the model given by the SM. If you have clear and distinct formation of the sounds in words, chances are that you will have a profoundly positive effect on the person with whom you are working, and they will accurately *imitate* your speech sounds.

There are people with speaking difficulties who may not be able to clearly say the words that you are giving them. Remember, the speech-language pathologist is the person who has received specialized training for people with this problem. It is always prudent to work in coordination with a speech-language pathologist. This professional can be of invaluable assistance to those who have mild to profound speaking difficulties. It is always advisable to have a professional standing by who can answer any questions you may have, or mentor you during the language stimulation phase and after discharge from formalized speech language therapy.

Dear Reader,

I would suggest that you complete the Speech Model Self-Evaluation Form, located at the end of this chapter, to the best of your ability. If you have any concerns related to your speaking ability, please ask up to three people you know to rate your speaking, using this same Self Evaluation Sheet. An SM should be rated at 3s and 4s for all of the questions. It is vital for a person with a communication difficulty to have a good speech model who represents all five of the above categories. Of course, the SM should also be patient, kind, loving, firm, persistent, and determined to use these methods.

Mark

markittleman@makerockstalk.com

The Third Ittle Principle — Speed

One of the fundamental principles I find so very important is that of speed in learning. Those of us who have normal hearing and brains can usually learn something quickly, but those with congenital or acquired speech and language problems may need to be approached with a simpler task they can readily achieve (principle #1), and they must also be approached with clarity (principle #2) by the SM. Another important principle is *speed of presentation*. If you present words to the SM simply, clearly, and *slowly,* the chances will be higher that the PCD will imitate them accurately. The two major factors I typically have to address with caregivers are simplicity and speed. Caregivers are accustomed to speaking at their normal speed, which includes an average number of words each time they say something. It will take some learning and repetition for them to simplify what they say to the PCD in few words at very slow speeds. It would be like asking you to drive at 45 miles per hour on a super highway. You are not accustomed to it, and it would make many of you initially uncomfortable.

For the caregiver this whole process is also like therapy for you. You have never been asked to simplify your speaking or to say it slowly with a marked separation between each word, such as when you talk to the PCD. Not only will this be a totally different experience for the PCD, but it will also be challenging for you. Expect some *moments* with this, but you will work through them.

The Fourth Ittle Principle — Stepping into the World of the Person with the Communication Difficulty

For you to have a real impact on the person you are stimulating, you must learn to enter the world of the PCD and find out who they are. That includes assessing what is important to them. Find out what they value as it pertains to family, life, and their specific communication difficulty. You must take the time to figure out what is relevant or irrelevant to the PCD. Make sure you ask them why they are seeking your services and what they want to improve upon. Listen to what they are saying so that you don't end up doing what YOU think is necessary. Make sure you consider what the PCD wants to accomplish in the therapeutic relationship. Then, when you know what is important to them, you can design your therapy to address their specific wants and needs just like a seamstress or a tailor designs or fits a dress or a suit.

One of my clients was a gentleman who was a "foodie." He loved food and liked to buy, prepare, and eat it. He also liked fine wines and beers. Often, as we were helping him regain his power to speak, we would name the kinds of beers that he liked and assign an adjective to each one (good beer, brown ale; stout beer; pilsner beer; etc.). He also loved to cook, and he and his wife would always experiment with new wines and ways to prepare food. Therefore our language stimulation included one and two word responses at the start of therapy. (The things he had in his refrigerator, and the different wines he liked: red, white, rose', champagne, and Riunite; dry, not sweet, etc.) He loved seafood, and we talked about crab, lobster, scallops, and a host of foods from the sea. To me it is critical that you consider what the PCD values and include those words, phrases, and sentences into your language stimulation. It will be exciting for them and for you. It will be far superior to the generic, boring materials that are taken from therapy notebooks.

Remember this: *Where there is interest there is mental attention. Mental attention is therefore related to how much interest your PCD has in the subject at hand.* You will learn new things through your conversations and then you can apply them to your own life. My friend (the way I see each patient) would often bring me samples of things that he thought I would like. We would then talk about that within the sentence length and complexity that he could readily say. Remember that speech and language is not static. It constantly changes in relation to the topic discussed. You will learn to discuss interesting topics in a structure in which the PCD can succeed. I cannot stress that point enough.

The other golden statement here is that when you approach a subject of personal interest with the PCD, the chances of more spontaneous speech are exponentially higher. When we talk about things that interest us, it is fun and stimulating and time distorts. You can learn to do therapy and not even realize you are doing it once you understand the structure and language complexity/ sentence length that is appropriate for each PCD. This knowledge will help you ask questions that will trigger a successful response. That will take a bit of practice, but you will achieve that!

The Fifth Ittle Principle — The Power is the Question

One of the underlying principles in the successful stimulation of speech and language is the proper utilization of a *simple question to stimulate speech*. The *question* by whomever asks it is inviting the other person to ponder an idea (think) and then to respond or communicate back to the one who asked with an answer. Therefore, if we are to engage people in speaking, we must pose questions since they are *open invitations to speak*. Embedded deeply within the question is the **gold of speaking**: the *vocabulary, grammar, and syntax* needed by the person who will be answering the question. If the question is posed with clarity, the underlying *articulation and pronunciation* of those words are also available for the PCD to duplicate. If you are going to help others with speaking, your speech when communicating must be *loud enough, simple, clear, and said at a speed that can be easily heard, understood, and remembered.*

Any person receiving stimulation for speech and language must be approached with respect, dignity, and courtesy. Occasionally, mistakes are made in speech therapy by well-meaning clinicians who expect the PCD to repeat prepared phrases or sentences. In some cases, that method may be the treatment of choice; however, that is not the way human interaction works. If we are to be courteous, we must ASK. *Asking* with a question is inviting the PCD into an interaction.

I believe the stimulation of speech and language follows the ways of learning first postulated by the great teachers of humanity, including Socrates and Plato. Socratic questioning is a commonly used tool in a wide range of discussions or what we may refer to as conversation and is a type of pedagogy. A series of questions are asked not only to draw individual answers, but also to encourage fundamental insight into the issue at hand. Remember what Wepman stated, that *thought stimulates language*. Wepman believed that we as SMs can stimulate words by *asking questions that stimulate thought.*

This is what happens in true speech and language stimulation. It is not having a person repeat common phrases or expressions, but engaging the thinking of the person through questioning that may be open ended or it may have the answer embedded within, which then gives the receiver of the question the voice, words, grammar, syntax, and answer to the question. This in turn provides the PCD with a feeling of achievement. And as the Socratic method implies, the answering of a question then leads the questioner to further related questions *of interest.*

The key to this method of interaction involves a conversation that necessitates posing questions, listening, language formulation and expression of speech and language. One of the interesting points to understand here is that this method is nothing new and has been around for centuries as it pertains to *pedagogy.* In early Greek times, a slave would be assigned to his master's child and supervise the instruction of his master's son. This necessitated taking the child to the school or a gym, looking after him and carrying his equipment (i.e., music instruments or anything which pertained to the education of that child). This concept is still practiced today especially relating to the parent, spouse, or caregiver of the PCD.

The Sixth Ittle Principle — The Use of Bombardment Within *The Teaching of Talking* Method

When you become proficient with the question and answer method for the stimulation of single words, you will find there are numerous other ways to stimulate language that include the fundamental principles of *auditory, visual, and motor bombardment*. *Visual bombardment* refers to presenting the word on a computer screen or piece of paper in printed or pictorial form, and stimulating single word speaking numerous times to impress the word in printed form to the visual system. *Auditory bombardment* refers to the word as it is perceived by the hearing mechanism over and over again, and *motor programming* describes the repetition of motor movements in speaking such as those needed to say the word "diadochokinesis." Practice saying this word now, and you will get the idea of motor programming: (die ae dah ko kah 'nee sis), which will lead to motor memory.

Children who are excellent spellers have been shown to have a "picture memory" of the word in printed form, and actually look at the word in their minds and recite each letter! The same concept of modeling the word (hearing-auditory memory), typing or writing it in large letters (motor + visual memory), and then asking the PCD to repeat the word with speaking (motor memory), works just as well when teaching someone to talk. In time, when the PCD recalls a word that he or she wishes to say, the visual image of the written word, and the sound memory of how it should sound, and motor movement of the spoken word, will likely come back to the PCD, and they will be able to speak the word from any preferred channel or all simultaneous channels of memory.

Auditory and motor bombardment is having the PCD *hear* and *speak* the word several times, such as in *Embedded Questions*, so that it will likely become learned as a sound bite file in the brain. In this instance, when the PCD recalls a word that may be in the auditory memory (from hearing it numerous times within *Embedded Questions*), he or she hears the word spoken from the sound memory and simultaneously says the word, since it was inputted into both auditory and motor memory. The probability that the PCD will speak the word is usually much better when it is programmed through the use of auditory bombardment within *Embedded Questions* and *Tell Me Phrases,* and repeated in spoken words.

The trick is to use all three ways of bombardment in the presentation of a word or phrase — letting the PCD *hear* the model, *see* the model and *say* the model numerous times. That will facilitate memory much faster than many of the traditional methods of speech therapy. These methods can be used with individuals or groups of individuals with communication difficulties. Schuell[10] originally

---

10   H. M. Schuell, J. J. Jenkins, and E. Jiminez-Pabon, Aphasia in Adults (New York, NY: Harper and Row, 1964); H. M. Schuell, V. Carroll, and B. S. Street, "Clinical Treatment of Aphasia," Journal of Speech and Hearing Disorders, 1955, 20, 43-53; and C. M. Scott, Editor's Note, Journal of Speech and Hearing Disorders, 42.

made significant contributions to the aphasia literature when she stressed intensive auditory stimulation in speech and language rehabilitation. Joseph Duffy and Carl Coelho in Chapey, 2001,[11] confirmed and expanded Schuell's approach and emphasized the necessity of using input from all modalities contributing to speech and language learning. The Teaching of Talking uses all sensory input modalities for speech including hearing, vision, and motor programming.

People who have aphasia of the *Broca's type* can imitate words, but have difficulty initiating speech. These language stimulation methods should be very helpful in assisting the PCD to utter speech with the cues you give them; and then with time, the likelihood is that they will be able to say the words they wish without your assistance.

Review

1. ***Make it Easy.*** Speak slowly, loudly, and use short, common words.
2. ***Emphasize Clarity.*** If you are going to model speech, then your speech must be clear and distinct, with proper formation of the sounds in words. You must demonstrate correct articulation, pronunciation, grammar, and sentence structure. Use repetition of single words, phrases, and sentences to build speech and language skills.
3. ***Speed.*** Model the optimum speed of speaking, which is slow enough for the PCD to hear the word or sound they are trying to imitate and then to pronounce that word or sound correctly. It is difficult for both the SM and the PCD to adjust their rate of speech, but doing so will limit the difficulty the PCD has been encountering in speaking.
4. ***Step into the PCD's World.*** The SM must take time to get to know who the PCD is: identify their specific speaking difficulty, find out who they are, what they value, and what they enjoy doing. The best way to get someone to talk is to ask them a question (invite them to talk) about something they know a lot about and have an intense interest in.
5. ***The Power is the Question.*** Questions are open invitations to speak. With the proper use of a simple question, the PCD will be successful duplicating the words the SM models.
6. ***Use of Bombardment.*** Use all three ways of bombardment when possible in the presentation of a word or phrase—letting the PCD hear, see, and say the model numerous times to facilitate memory.

---

11   Anonymous, Language Intervention Strategies in Adult Aphasia, 4th ed., (Baltimore: Lippincott Williams & Wilkins, April 15, 2001).

We should always approach people with speaking difficulties with respect, courtesy and dignity.

Speech Model Self-Evaluation Form

Name:_____Date: _____

Please circle how you would describe your speech in the questions below using the following rating scale:

4:     All of the time
3:     Most of the time
2:     Some of the time
1:     Not very often

1. My speech is loud enough to be clearly understood?
    1   2   3   4
2. The speed of my speech is slow enough for others to understand?
    1   2   3   4
3. The sounds in my words are clearly heard by others.
    1   2   3   4
4. My speech is intelligible or understandable to others.
    1   2   3   4
5. My voice is clear and strong.
    1   2   3   4

Please make comments below, regarding your speech, relating to each question:

Loudness:

Speed of Speaking:

Sounds of Speech:

Understandability of my speech:

Voice Clarity:

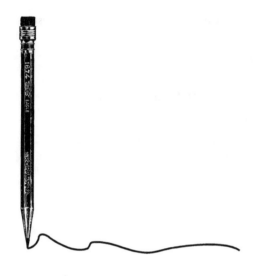

Getting Down to
the Actual Work

The stimulation of language can be accomplished in many ways. The method I usually use is the *Questioning Method*. With severe to profound speech and language difficulty, it is often beneficial to start stimulation at the individual's expressive speech and language level. If the person is not speaking with any degree of clarity and cannot be understood due to an inability to initiate speech, it would be wise to start at the *Single-Word Level,* which will enable you and the PCD to get comfortable and coordinated as a team. The person who is stimulating the speech and language is the SM, and the person with the communication difficulty is the PCD. The SM and PCD become *partners in communication*. The PCD becomes a *mirror* of the SM. When stimulating the PCD, the SM must be able to set it up in such a way that the PCD's mouth, tongue, lips, and palate will move at the same time as the SM's. They move in *unison*. The reason for starting at the *Single-Word Level* is to have the SM and PCD learn to coordinate the *steps of speaking*, very much like coordinating a dance step. The two people must start simply, in harmony and synchronicity with one another.

Set Up

Set up so that the PCD sits directly across from you, the SM, at approximately three to five feet (a little bit farther away than where you would sit if you were looking in a mirror). Remember, when you are sitting across from the PCD, it is as if you are looking at yourself in the mirror. Make sure you are looking directly into the eyes of the PCD and that they are, likewise, looking into yours. By maintaining eye contact with one another, you can be relatively assured that you will have the full attention of the PCD. This is the *connection* that must be established at the start of *The Teaching of Talking*.

Not long ago, I was working with a gentleman in a wheelchair. His chair was not in direct relation to me and must have been off by about 20 degrees. As I was working with him, he was not looking directly into my eyes. For some reason, I became uncomfortable. I soon realized that we were not lined up eye-to-eye and nose-to-nose, creating a feeling of disconnection between us. When I moved his chair 20 degrees to the right, I immediately felt the connection established.

I cannot emphasize enough the importance of lining up eye-to-eye and nose-to-nose, as if you were looking into a full-length mirror. You will notice an improved connection and an ability to work more readily with one another.

Imitation

Start this imitation task by moving all of the structures of your mouth, tongue, lips, or head in one specific movement. Let the PCD know that you want him or her to be a mirror image of you, to move exactly as you do and at the same time. That is how dancers do it. They dance in synchrony, "as one." You also want a setting where the PCD mirrors your face, mouth, lip, and tongue movements when the two of you are working in unison. For instance, when you are sitting across from each other, pucker your lips, smile, open your mouth, and close it. Stick out your tongue, move it to the right and left, elevate the tongue tip and try to touch it to your nose; then move the tongue tip and point it down towards the ground. Curl the tongue back towards your throat so that the tongue tip is pointing towards the *uvula*. Nod your head for "yes" and shake your head for "no." This is a critical step because it establishes whether or not the PCD can move in unison with you. Once it can be established that the individual you are working with can *mirror* basic nonspeaking movements, you can then move on to say individual vowels, sounds, and words with the same speed, melody, tone, and manner. In articulation therapy, there is a fundamental principle called *placement* and *production*. Before an individual can model what is being said, they must be able to place their mouth, tongue, and lips in the same position as the SM, and they must be able to clearly imitate the movement and sound that is being presented. The single *vowel, consonant-vowel cluster*, or word must be imitated by the PCD. This will give you, as the SM, an idea of how well the individual can imitate.

In speech therapy methodology, the more easily one can imitate what is being said, the better the prognosis for improvement with stimulation. Therefore, if you find that the PCD is not able to imitate vowels (a, e, i, o, oo), consonants (p, b, m, w, s, t, d, n, l, sh, f, v, th, etc.), consonant-vowel combinations (bay, be, bye, boh, boo, may, me, my, mow, moo), or single words (hi, bye, yes, no, now, water, me, you), they may have a problem referred to as either *acquired* or *developmental apraxia of speech*. An acquired apraxia of speech can affect a person at any age, although it most typically occurs in adults. It is caused by damage to the parts of the brain that are involved in speaking, resulting in an impairment of speech. It may occur as the result of a stroke, head injury, tumor, or other illness affecting the brain. An acquired apraxia of speech may occur together with muscle weakness, affecting speech production (such as articulation errors and *dysarthria*). Concurrent language difficulties such as aphasia may also occur due to central nervous system damage. The individual with apraxia of speech has marked difficulty voluntarily moving the speech structures. We will not be covering therapy methods for profound apraxia of speech in this text since it requires instruction and familiarity with the sounds of speech or phonetics. This text is more concerned with the *formulation of intelligible speech and language with those who can generally articulate the sounds of speech*. The author has plans for a follow-up text which will address apraxia of speech and how to help those who have difficulty saying speech sounds.

For the purpose of this chapter regarding the stimulation of speech and language, we are going to assume that the person with whom you are working can say simple vowels and words if you give them a slow, clear example. In order for you to become an accomplished stimulator of speaking in *The Teaching of Talking* method, you will become adept at utilizing questions to facilitate spoken single words. Remember, these words should be pronounced slowly and with distinct, full voice and volume so the PCD can hear the sounds and words clearly.

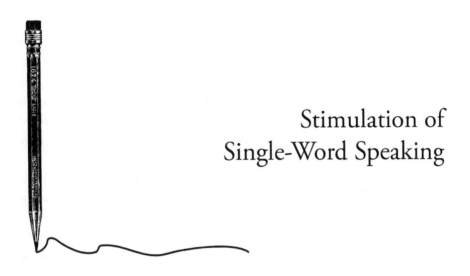

Stimulation of
Single-Word Speaking

The following methods of speech and language stimulation are typically successful with individuals who have mild to profound speaking difficulties. You will find that many of these methods will stimulate speech because we embed the target word that we want spoken within the question asked.

The Embedded Question for the Stimulation of the Single Words "Yes" and "No"

The first objective a clinician should have when beginning speech therapy with those who have lost the ability to speak, or with those who are not speaking, is to determine the PCD's ability to understand and use either nonverbal or verbal forms of the words "yes" and "no." Many speech-language pathologists have difficulty with this concept because people with speaking difficulties may confuse "yes" and "no" when they listen to others or while they are speaking. However, I do not think "yes" and "no" have to be difficult for the speech clinician or caregiver, provided that they are observant.

Calibration in the Use of "Yes" and "No"

As a speech-language pathologist, I have never been all that concerned about the use of "yes" and "no." I know that for some PCDs, the concept is easy to learn with stimulation, which we will soon review. For others, it may be difficult. I never spend time on a behavior that doesn't get me the "best bang for the buck." I want to begin with speech behaviors that can be readily improved upon and return to the ones that are not amenable to stimulation at a later time in the clinical process.

When I studied behavioral therapy in the 1980s, gurus like Richard Bandler and John Grinder were developing a new way of helping people change behavior. Inspired by them, I decided to learn whatever I could to help those who were resistant to change. Their therapy was called "*Neuro-Linguistic Programming*,"[12] and from it I learned many distinctions about behavioral change and what was necessary in order to help people do what they seemingly could not do by themselves. In particular, I learned how to read the communications of others by listening to voice and tonality, watching specific mannerisms of the body, and listening for the words people used.

Calibration is the ability to judge by observation, specifically for repeated behaviors. In this conversation, it is a form of measurement to determine the PCD's standard nonverbal responses to "yes" and "no."

If you want to calibrate a physical *Yes/No* response, you might ask someone ten questions to which you know the answers are unmistakably "yes", such as:

- Is it morning?
- Is it Monday?
- Are you married?
- Do you live in a house?
- Are you a man?

While you are asking these questions, observe the PCD's facial and bodily responses to the "yes" questions. You should find that the person who is being asked the questions will display a consistent bodily response for "yes." It might be a nodding of the head, closing of the eyes, other movements, or gestures that will be consistent. (As an aside,

---

12   WebFinance, Inc., BusinessDictionary.com, s.v. "neuro-linguistic programming," accessed: February 13, 2012, http://www.businessdictionary.com/definition/neuro-linguistic-programming-NLP.html.

I suggest practicing this with normal-speaking persons before you attempt it on someone who has a speaking difficulty.)

Next, calibrate their bodily movements and gestures for "no." Ask questions that you know should get a "no" response and simultaneously observe the movement of the head, eyes, nose, and mouth. You should, after a number of "no" questions, begin to recognize a pattern for what a "no" looks like in automatic gestural or nonverbal communication.

Beginning clinicians often set "yes" and "no" as the early goals of speech therapy. Most married couples will ask each other questions and know the answers before the other verbally responds. They have subconsciously calibrated their mate and can just watch the face, bodily mannerisms, and listen to the voice tonality to pick up the answer. Expert trial lawyers can tell with relative consistency whether a person is telling the truth by calibrating tonal, facial, and eye movements.

The same holds true with children and their mothers. Often, the mother can look at her child when a question is posed and know the answer by observing the child's *physiology,* or their physical, nonverbal movements. The ability to subconsciously calibrate "yes" and "no" adds great value to a speech pathologist's clinical work repertoire. Caregivers would also be wise to pay attention to the *physiology* of "yes" and "no" responses. These nonverbal gestures are instinctual for the PCD, and we must learn to read them.

Using Embedded Questions to Facilitate the Use of "Yes"

I like things simple. I had learning problems as a child and am profoundly aware of and respect the learning challenges of others. Simplification and repetition is how I always had to approach learning myself, so I use the same methods when teaching others. Later on in this text, you will read about my "tying your shoes" approach to speech therapy. Perhaps my own learning style has contributed to my ability to help many people with developmental or acquired neurologically related difficulties.

If you want a person to learn to actually *speak* the words "yes" and "no," it may be challenging. It is for this reason that I have to teach specific speech behaviors sequentially. Since I am not known for my multitasking ability, I rarely use it in my approach to therapy. Multitasking, as defined by Merriam-Webster, is the performance of multiple tasks at one time and requires a certain level of higher cognitive ability that people with communication difficulties may not possess at the time of treatment.

Therefore, if I wanted to stimulate a verbal response for "yes" and "no," I would first work on each concept and make sure that the PCD comprehends and expresses the task correctly. For instance, when working on the first goal of getting a PCD to answer a "yes" question to 99%, I would start out with only "yes" questions. That is where I went wrong as a new clinician, by asking both "yes" and "no" questions in the same clinical interaction. By the end of the time allotted, we were both extremely frustrated! Having learned from my early clinical mistakes, I want to give you an example of how the dialogue would sound and look today.

Remember to calibrate the "yes" and "no" responses — if you can observe them, that is — as long as the PCD with whom you are working does actually have a consistent way to express "yes" and "no" with face, eyes, facial features, or mannerisms. There may be some low-functioning PCDs who are unable to express "yes" and "no" responses consistently by their physiology.

Example

SM: Hello, James. Are you sitting down?

PCD: (James nods while squinting and smiling.)

SM: Now, James, you are a man, right?
(A look of surprise; then a laugh from me like I am teasing him, which I am. I like humor and surprise!)

SM: And you are a man, right?

PCD: (Nodding, squinting, and smiling)

SM: And you are married, right?

PCD: (Nodding, squinting, and smiling)

SM: And she is your wife? (Clinician points at woman sitting to his left.)

SM: She's your wife, right?

PCD: (Nodding, squinting, and smiling)

SM: Any kids?

PCD: (Nodding, squinting, and smiling)

At this point in the interview, I have calibrated a number of responses that seem consistent. I can either cull for more nonverbal responses to "yes" questions, or I can begin stimulating a verbal "yes" at this point.

I also have a curve ball that I can throw if I want to know if the PCD has a nonverbal "no."

Example

SM: Now James, I heard your wife's name is Lucretia (or some other off-the-wall name).

(I sometimes do this just to see if I can get a rise out of the person and thus get a truly accurate response for "no." If I get a good "no" response, I might ask the PCD a few other "off-the-wall" questions that would be both humorous and unexpected. If I get a similar physiology for "no" with unexpected "no" questions, then I feel relatively sure that I have the "yes" and "no" calibrated.)

SM: I heard the two of you were newlyweds, right?

PCD: (Shaking head with smirk and wrinkled forehead)

(In this case, they had been married for forty years! By asking questions that are totally unexpected, you can often get a more accurate determination of true competence with a nonverbal "yes" or "no" response.)

One of the things I was taught early in my career was that *receptive* language always precedes *expressive* language. I used to agree with this idea, but now I realize there are few hard and fast rules to human response and behavior. I say that because some people with communication difficulties sometimes learn things first by saying a word and then developing the idea of the concept cognitively. So, I do not think it is always necessary to stay with the receptive language or comprehension factors in exercises, or in "yes" or "no" drills before stimulating the actual spoken words.

If I am not able to calibrate a "yes" or "no" response nonverbally, it could mean that attempting expression of these concepts in speech might be difficult — or maybe not. I then choose whether to continue with the stimulation of "yes" and "no" in speech.

Stimulation of "Yes" and "No" in Speaking

SM: Now, is your name "James"?

PCD: (Nodding, squinting, and smiling)

SM: YES?

PCD: (Nodding, squinting, and smiling)

SM: Tell me: YES!

PCD: YES!

> *ALL CAPS will be used in these examples to denote the word(s) the SM is modeling and the word(s) actually spoken by the PCD.

SM: Is she your wife?
PCD: (Nodding, squinting)
SM: Tell me: YES!
PCD: YES!
SM: Did she drive? (to the office/clinic)
PCD: (Nodding, squinting)
SM: YES? (Upward inflection to my voice)
PCD: (Nodding)
SM: Say: YES!
PCD: YES.

The questioning can continue in this manner, asking all kinds of interesting questions to which you, the SM, already know the answer, especially if you have a case history or face sheet at your disposal. Caregivers or family members may be at an advantage since they already know interesting, personal questions to ask.

You could ask "yes" questions that pertain to their appearance, age, birthday, address, children, occupation, and the like. If you have calibrated their "yes" and "no" responses, you will often know whether the answers are correct. I do my best to ask only questions to which I know the answer. Occasionally, throughout the session, I throw in another *Yes/No* question to confirm that they are still using the same gestures for "yes" and "no."

In this example, I recommend staying with the "yes" questions until you are sure that the PCD can easily answer them by saying "yes" exclusively. By exclusively, I mean that the SM can observe the nonverbal "yes" and then stimulate the proper word "yes" in speech, using an *embedded question* or *Tell Me: YES* or *Say: YES* cue. I would not be concerned about whether they got it right each time without cues. However, I would make sure they got it right each time through my questioning and cueing with *Tell me: YES* or *Say: YES,* so there is no *negative practice.*

In learning, we want correct responses consistently, since that will lead to more rapid carry-over at an unconscious or automatic level. If a clinician is stimulating "yes" and "no," and the PCD is making correct and incorrect responses, there is *negative practice,* which is the potential to practice saying the wrong answer. That is why I consistently prompt with the *Tell Me: YES* and *Say: YES* cues, so that each time I ask the question, they get it right! This facilitates learning!

Once the "yes" is established, the next step is to work on the "no" with the methods described above. Listen closely to the PCD. The mistake most clinicians and caregivers make is that they try to get a PCD to answer the *Yes/No* questions right away without cues. Please! Cue with *Tell Me: (Yes/No)* or *SAY: (Yes/No)* cues so that they always use the word correctly without negative practice. In time, they will surprise you and answer your question without cues. The way to achieve consistent learning is to expect consistent responses with few, if any, errors. That is why you will want to facilitate *Yes/No* answers at 100% accuracy in your goals. Your PCD can achieve those results in your training if you just make sure that you're feeding them the cues. Then, before long, voilà!

The Embedded Question for Nouns and Verbs (Single Word)

A question always requires an answer. Therefore, *Embedded Questions* that are used in this therapy to elicit single words, phrases, or sentences always require a *Yes/No* response from the PCD.

When you are able to calibrate and stimulate the PCD to actually say "yes" and "no," you can move on to the stimulation of single words, made up of nouns, verbs, adjectives, and prepositions. Remember that the *Embedded Question* is one of the foundation blocks of *The Teaching of Talking* method to speech and language stimulation, especially for moderate to profound speaking difficulties.

Therefore, if I am going to request an answer to my question, I must first ascertain whether the PCD's answer is a "yes" or a "no." Once I know the answer to my question, I am then in a position as a speech model to take the PCD to the next step of therapy, which is the speaking of nouns and verbs, since a noun and verb are necessary to express a complete thought. Insert a noun or verb into the following question to get the PCD to speak a single word.

Example

SM: Do you want milk?
PCD: (Shakes head)
SM: NO?
PCD: NO.

Nouns:
If the answer is affirmative, it would be a different interaction.

Example
Three-repetition model for those who require more stimulation

SM: Do you want milk?
PCD: (Nods head)
SM: YES?
PCD: YES.
SM: Tell me: YES.
PCD: YES.
SM: So you want MILK? (1)
PCD: (Nods head)
SM: YES?
PCD: YES.
SM: Tell me: MILK. (2)
PCD: MILK. (3)

The answer should be forthcoming since you have used mild *auditory bombardment*[13] with the person you are stimulating. Auditory bombardment focuses on stimulating words or language by repeating sounds, words, phrases, and sentences. This work was pioneered by Schuell[14] and is based on the idea that repeating words at a volume that can be easily heard by the PCD helps in language learning and expression of those with aphasia. For the PCD who is not able to imitate easily, one can add a few additional repetitions of the modeled word, which will again bombard the person with the key word you wish them to say.

Seven-repetition model for those who require more stimulation
Example

SM: Do you want MILK? (1)
PCD: UHM UHM.
SM: YES?

13   Betsy Partin Vinson, Essentials for Speech-Language Pathologists (San Diego, CA: Singular Publishing Group, 2001).
14   Hildred Schuell, James J. Jenkins, Edward Jiménez-Pabón, Aphasia in Adults: Diagnosis, Prognosis, and Treatment, 4th ed. (Hoeber Medical Division, Harper & Row, 1969).

PCD: YES.
SM: Oh, MILK? (2)
PCD: UHM.
SM: YES?
PCD: YES.
SM: Tell me: MILK! (3) (elevate pitch on key word)
PCD: MILK.
SM: Great. Tell me: MILK! (4) (elevate pitch again)
PCD: MILK.
SM: You can really say MILK! (5)
SM: I love how you say MILK! (6)
SM: Tell me: MILK! (7)
PCD: MILK.

The key here is repetition and using your voice as a penetrative force, so that he or she can repeat it in a way that is easy and prevents frustration.

The exercise for the SM is to practice stimulating nouns with your PCD until this becomes second nature to both of you. In the examples above, you are given a simple, *three-repetition* and *seven-repetition strategy*. In many cases, this will be enough stimulation to obtain the desired response of the single word. If it is *not*, then remember to use auditory bombardment with more repetition, cueing *Tell Me Phrases* and increased vocal loudness and emphasis until the word is said. The PCD may be able to say the word more easily if the word is also presented simultaneously in large letters. You may find that small, single syllable words (I, me, you, night, day, eat, go, TV, etc.) are easier to stimulate.

If you do not achieve success with the above strategy, it may be due to numerous factors. Please keep your voice *loud enough* to have a penetrating effect. Make sure you *say the word slowly* and that you *articulate each sound within the word clearly*.

 Write down the important items (nouns) in the PCD's home and their location in each room. It is important that you do this thoroughly.

Start in the places where the PCD spends time. If it is in the bedroom, note all of the objects there: bed, blankets, pillows; drawers and what is in each one; pictures on the wall; what is on each bedside table and in the drawers. List the items and objects in the bathroom, including the fixtures, sink, toilet, shower, bidet; and what is on the counter, including the toothbrushes, soap, and so on. Don't forget the medicine cabinet, the items beneath the sink, and the contents of each cabinet and closet, especially if the PCD may need to request these items.

Be sure to list everything that can be found in the kitchen, including each item in the refrigerator, as well as the cabinets, drawers, and pantry. Keep a list for each room in the house and for the garage, if applicable, and organize the items by their specific location.

Don't miss anything, including what is in the recreation areas, such as games, CDs, and DVDs. Include the places the PCD goes: the supermarket, and the items you buy there; the places you shop, and what is purchased there; the bank, and all the words associated with banking, such as *deposit* and *withdrawal* and the denominations of money that are deposited or withdrawn on a regular basis. Also include the names of coins and paper money.

If you go to restaurants, list each one that the PCD likes to visit, as well as their favorite entrées. There may be certain food preferences they order at various restaurants. One gentleman I know, who goes out to eat often, likes Italian, Chinese, Mexican, Indian, and, of course, fast food restaurants if he is in a hurry to get somewhere in town, such as doctor appointments. He likes eggplant parmesan and spaghetti, pizza, ravioli, and lasagna at the Italian place; chicken soup, burritos, and chicken enchiladas with a cold Corona or Modelo at the Mexican place; and coffee, a Big Mac, and fries occasionally at McDonalds! You could literally list hundreds of items for this PCD.

It is best to go through the house room by room to note items, or sit down and mentally go through each one. Imagine you are going to each of the places you visit, listing the vocabulary for each establishment you frequent. The more custom-made the list is, the better.

I was recently working with a gentleman who had an iPad. His caregiver took literally dozens of pictures each day and imported them into his iPad by category. By this, I mean that he would photograph the bathroom, starting with the fixtures, then move on to every item in every drawer and cabinet. He would classify the items and create a picture file of everything, such as what was in the medicine cabinet and what was in the shower, including the shampoo, razor, conditioner, and soap.

In taking photographs of specific areas in the bathroom, he created a "shower file" with its items; the "medicine chest" file had its items, and the "under the sink" file had its own. Although each word was stimulated for the PCD using the actual item within the activities of daily living, each one of the words was also photographed and placed in the photographic section of the iPad so it could be accessed, if needed, by pressing on the photo album icon. Specific files (shower, medicine chest, closet, under the sink, Italian Restaurant, Mexican Restaurant, McDonalds, etc.) could be easily located by the PCD by touching the actual picture file icon of those locations or places, which would then open, revealing all of the contents within.

If you have word processing software, you can use it to alphabetize the words as they apply to each room.

> I want to emphasize that *The Teaching of Talking* approach prides itself on stimulating the word, phrase, or sentence in the context of the situation when *the opportunity or necessity is present*. The reason for putting all of the words in a list, photo album, digital file, or iPad application is to facilitate the PCD expressing what they may want, either by pointing, or pointing and speaking when they are away from the specific context and when it is immediately necessary for the PCD to express a desire or need.

Some caregivers print the word in an extra-large font underneath each picture, which also helps the PCD say it more readily. They won't have to play the "100 questions game," where the caregiver or family member has to keep questioning the PCD until the concept of what the PCD wants is identified. We would prefer words to be practiced in real time in the real situation, rather than "practicing" lists or photographs of words from a notebook or device; but the notebooks or picture books can come in handy in a pinch when the PCD has something he or she wants to say! There is nothing worse for any human being than to have an idea or word that needs to be expressed but not have immediate access to its expression. Notebooks or picture books can provide an alternate way for the PCD to identify and express an urgent need when words allude them.

You could choose some of the most important words from the list provided below, but I strongly encourage you to use the words that pertain to the PCD, where they live, and within their world. Then review and practice the *three-repetition* and *seven-repetition* model previously reviewed to stimulate these words.

○				○	
bath	pee	coffee	eggs	milk	juice
pills	knife	spoon	fork	toast	jam
phone	cup	shoe	pet	bank	doctor
car	cake	bed	light	TV	phone
heat	toy	dog	door	hot	A/C
coke	tea	water	cookie	lunch	soda
bowl	soup	cold	pants		

Nouns and *verbs* are powerful words in the English language. When combined (noun +verb), we have a sentence. For children who are not talking, or for adults who have lost the ability to express language due to brain injury, I like to start speech and language stimulation at the single-word level. When a person is competent in the expression of single words, with or without cues, the SM can then, *and only then,* move on to word pairs, phrases, and sentences, depending on the severity of the speaking difficulty.

Additional Practice
Three-repetition model for single word nouns or verbs
Verbs

SM: Want to GO? (1)
PCD: Hm mmm.
SM: YES?
PCD: YES.
SM: Okay. Tell me: GO! (2) (Say the word "GO" with increased loudness and upward vocal inflection.)
PCD: GO!

SM: Tell me again: GO!
PCD: GO!

If the PCD has difficulty saying any word or specific speech sound, such as the initial "g," you could choose a different word to stimulate; or, if the word is important and can be understood by the listener, go ahead and stimulate it. You may not, at first, get accurate articulation, but if you can understand the word spoken, accept it and do not beat a dead horse for perfection.

Successive approximation in speech therapy is a concept whereby you initially accept the way a word is said by the PCD, so long as you understand it, even though it may not be perfect. The thought is that with time and repetition, the word will be uttered more accurately as the motor speech mechanism gets accustomed to saying words again. With a good SM saying the word, the PCD will probably surprise you as the sounds within the words improve. In the above example, there were three opportunities for auditory bombardment. If that did not get the job done, you may want to increase the repetition as demonstrated in the previous example of stimulating nouns.

Keep in mind that at any sign of significant *frustration*, it is best to remember that frustration is the nonfulfillment of some need or wish, and occurs when the task presented is too difficult. *Your* job is to make the task *easier.* Use an easier word if the individual is having too much difficulty with the one you have selected. Remember that the single syllable word will usually be easier to stimulate and say than the word or words with more than one syllable. (*Example:* "pee" versus "urinate," or "TV" versus "television," or "Dee" versus "Delores.")

Example
Seven repetition model for those who require more stimulation
SM: Want to GO? (1)
PCD: Hmm.
SM: YES?
PCD: YES.
SM: Tell me: GO! (2)
PCD: Mmm.
SM: YES?
PCD: YES.
SM: Say: GO! (3) (pause and wait for response)

SM: Want to GO? (4) (pause and wait for response)
SM: Tell me: GO! (5) (pause and wait for response)
SM: And you say: GO! (6) (pause and wait for response)
SM: Tell me: GO! (7) (pause and wait for response)
PCD: GO!

In the above example, the SM exits the model as soon as the PCD responds with the single word. If the word is not forthcoming, the SM continues with the auditory bombardment *with questions and Tell Me Phrases* until the PCD expresses the desired word. Once the stimulated word is spoken, do your best to have it repeated numerous times to start programming memory. Remember to exit the strategy if the frustration mounts or if the word desired is too difficult.

 Now, add a list of commonly used verbs to your notebook or computer file. You may begin the list with the following words, but be sure to add verbs used by your PCD.

Now practice stimulating these verbs:

◯			◯	
go	drink	eat	walk	sleep
nap	see	shop	cut	mop
sit	watch	read	write	take
give	wash	brush	trim	wake
shave	play	clean	pee	hear
lie	lay	do	get	turn

Vocal bombardment will help facilitate the PCD to say the word more easily and automatically the next time. I would suggest that you have your PCD say the targeted single word five times if you are at the single word or multiple word level; and then periodically throughout the session, restimulate it with the same approach to questioning. By embedding the word desired into the short question, the SM serves up the word, which is simple for most PCDs to say. If it is relatively easy to say, there is no frustration, anger, or feeling of diminished self-worth. Our PCD should be successfully achieving the task we have set up.

It is vital that the PCD has extensive practice time saying words. In the beginning, your PCD may do better at the *Single-Word Level*. With time and mastery, you can expand to two words, phrases, or sentences of increasing length.

Practicing the What It Is© Method
Example

SM: I am going to describe myself, and you do the same; okay?
(Type in "OKAY" so PCD can see the word.)

SM: OKAY?

PCD: OKAY.

SM: I'm WELL. (Type or print WELL in large font simultaneously)

SM: Are you WELL?

PCD: WELL.

SM: I'm GOOD. (Type or print GOOD in large font simultaneously.)

SM: Are you GOOD?

PCD: Uh hmmm.

SM: YES?

PCD: YES.

SM: GOOD?

PCD: GOOD.

SM: I'm TIRED. (Type or print TIRED in large font simultaneously.)

SM: Are you TIRED?

PCD: Uh hmmm.

SM: YES?

PCD: YES.

SM: TIRED?

PCD: TIRED.

or

SM: I'M HOT! (Type or print HOT in large font simultaneously.)

SM: Are you HOT?

PCD: Uh hmmm.

SM: YES?

PCD: YES.

SM: HOT?

PCD: HOT.

Remember that with training, the PCD should automatically hear your question and see the visual cue from paper or computer, and respond appropriately in speech with the single word. You can feel free to stimulate nouns, verbs, and adjectives, or even prepositions; *whatever is appropriate within the conversation.*

Various therapeutic methods of speech and language stimulation suggest the utilization of intensive repetition and forced use all day, each and every day to help establish automatic speech.[15] We understand the role of repetition in any kind of learning. All of us can remember learning the addition and multiplication tables, The Lord's Prayer, or the alphabet. Silverman (LSVT)[16] suggests repeating a specific therapy word five times during stimulation. Going back to the previous models, it would be good to set a goal of at least five repetitions the first time you introduce a new target word, phrase, or sentence. This is how it might look and sound:

SM: I'm HUNGRY!

SM: Are you HUNGRY?

PCD: Uh hmmm.

SM: YES?

PCD: YES.

SM: HUNGRY?

PCD: HUNGRY!

SM: Great, HUNGRY. Can you tell me that again? HUNGRY! (still showing word cue on computer or paper)

PCD: HUNGRY!

SM: Great. Let's practice HUNGRY a few more times. What are you?

PCD: HUNGRY.

SM: Did you say HUNGRY?

PCD: HUNGRY!

SM: Great! Tell me one more time what you are!

PCD: HUNGRY!

---

15   Friedemann Pulvermuller, et al., "Constraint-Induced Therapy of Chronic Aphasia After Stroke," Stroke 32 (2001): 1621, accessed January 2012, http://stroke.ahajournals.org/content/32/7/1621. short.

16   "History of Lee Silverman Voice Treatment ," The National Center for Voice and Speech. accessed November 2011. http://www.ncvs.org/research/lsvt-history.html.

As you can see from the questions within the *What It Is©* Method, the conversation is very brief and to the point at the onset of treatment. The clinician or caregiver speaks slowly, with plenty of intensity, and emphasizing all the sounds within all words; the *model and the resultant speech required in response* is purposefully telegraphic. The PCD must be stimulated in conversation with simple speech to start talking. Think of the PCD as if they were the tortoise, as in the story of the Tortoise and the Hare. Those of us with normal speech and communication are like the hare, who can move at very fast speeds; but the PCD, if he is going to be included in the conversation, must be spoken to at his or her level of speaking ability. If the PCD speaks at a level of one or two words, it is prudent to stimulate their speaking from that level and help expand them first by one word, and then more as tolerated. What I am really stating here is this: *talk to them in the model that is appropriate for them.* If they are speaking in one or two words, so should you. Model what they can do and then expand by small increments, most likely a single word. With some you might be able to make more than a one-word expansion, perhaps to two words or more!

Alternate Choice

> If your PCD has been unable to speak but they can answer an *Alternate Choice Question*, this is a great place to start. It is very important to keep giving them *Alternate Choice Questions* in single words until this becomes second nature to you and them. Once it is second nature, then you can start to expand from the single word response.

I propose that speech stimulation can be easily and readily accomplished anywhere, and it is especially powerful when the PCD is stimulated in the context of the situation in which speech needs to be generated. *Choice* is important for all of us, and it is cordial and courteous to give our loved ones choices in communicative interactions. You should see a marked increase in the amount of speaking when people are given a *choice in the matter.* The key to this program, *The Teaching of Talking*, is your success in stimulating language in clear and concise utterances to the PCD, allowing them to hear unadulterated speech that is served up and presented to them in manageable bite-sized pieces that can be readily imitated. It is like the proverbial joke about the elephant: "How do you eat an elephant?" Like doing speech therapy, of course: "One bite at a time."

Example

SM:	Would you like COKE or WATER? (Remember to mark the key words with increased loudness and emphasis.)
PCD:	UH UM.
SM:	YES?
PCD:	YES.
SM:	COKE? ➔ or ➔ WATER?
	Arrows (➔), used in this text, indicate the SM should speak one word at a time, pausing between each word.
PCD:	WATER.

This method can be a lot of fun, as everyone loves to make choices, especially those who have difficulty speaking. By giving the PCD a choice and letting them hear the models of what you are offering, you are leaving the answer to the question up to them, while at the same time modeling the answer. It is also enjoyable for the PCD, because offering choices is a "giving activity," and will give them more opportunities to succeed with speaking tasks. This approach lends itself to increased speaking confidence, as the PCD is given the choice, requiring thought and expression. Accurate replies are *reinforcing,* and increase the likelihood of speaking performance.

How about another *Alternate Choice* opportunity for you to learn this very simple method?

Example

SM:	Want to go now or later?
PCD:	UH UM.

Whenever you do not receive an answer, ask the same question again, pausing a few seconds between each emphasized word.

SM:	NOW ➔ or ➔ LATER?
PCD:	NOW.

SM: Did you say "NOW?" (*Embedded Question*)
PCD: NOW.
SM: Yes. Very good! What did you say? (Checking immediate memory)
PCD: NOW!

Remember that when you complete the stimulation of a single word, word-pair, phrase, or sentence, have the PCD repeat it as often as is appropriate at the time and place, so it will become part of their automatic expressive *lexicon*.

The Phrase Completion

The *Phrase Completion Method* is another way to stimulate language. The SM says the start of the phrase and the PCD completes it. This method can be used anytime, anyplace, or anywhere, and should become second nature to the SM. If the PCD is unable to complete the phrases, this exercise may be too advanced. If so, go back to the other methods where the model is given in the *Embedded Question,* in an *Alternate Choice,* or through conversational statements that I refer to as *What It Is*© statements. Phrase completions are opportunities to stimulate speech and language. Why? Because they can also be used during activities of daily living (*ADLs*).

We know that in order to learn anything, it must be repeated over and over again. Why not repeat the speech and language utterance on a daily basis in the situation where the words "live?" That's what moms do when stimulating toddlers to talk. It is preferable to stimulate words within the context of those activities. You can readily turn this exercise into an *Embedded Question* if they are unable to complete the phrase. Depending upon the severity of the speaking difficulty, you may find that one or more methods may work best in the beginning. If that is true, stay with the method that works until such time as you choose something else to add to the mix of methods.

I am currently working with a woman who has been receiving speech therapy for about six weeks, and responds well to the *Embedded Question* model with a printed word cue. She loves that, and I will continue with this method until it is no longer necessary. You will find that the *Embedded Question* method will no longer be necessary with repeated practice. After a while, you will be able to just ask a question and get a single word, phrase, or complete sentence!

Example

Time to wake _____. (up)

Ready to get out of _____? (bed)

Want to take a _____ ? (pee, poop, etc.)

Brush your _____? (teeth, hair)

Dry yourself with the _____. (towel/washcloth)

Let's shave with the _____? (razor)

Put on your _____? (glasses, lipstick)

Put it under your _____. (arm/s)

Put on your _____? (cologne, perfume, aftershave)

> **(Make sure you have the item of clothing in your hand so they can see it.)**

Put on your _____. (underwear, panties, brief, etc.)

Put on your _____? (bra, blouse, shirt, pants, socks, shoes)

Put on the right/left_____. (sock)

Put on your right/left _____. (shoe)

Here is your _____. (cane, walker, etc.)

I'll get your _____. (wheelchair)

Want some hot _____? (coffee)

It's time for _____. (breakfast)

By plugging into your imagination, you can begin to think about phrases you might say. Be sure to stop right before the target word you are trying to get. If they cannot complete the phrase you have given them, remember to ask an *Embedded Question*: How about some hot_____? (coffee).

You could say out loud:

SM: Do you want coffee?

PCD: (Nods head)

SM: YES?

PCD: YES.

SM: Is it COFFEE you want?

PCD: COFFEE.

SM: You want COFFEE?

PCD: COFFEE.

Follow and actually do these procedures at every appropriate opportunity. Please do this from memory — no papers allowed after you have practiced this! If you have to, use a cheat sheet in the beginning; but after a while, you will want to have these methods in your automatic repertoire to stimulate talking. For the *Phrase Completion* model example, you are about to serve breakfast with the coffee, and the PCD can see the steaming cup and smell its aroma! You will get more consistent responses if you have the actual object. Let the PCD see it while stimulating the word, phrase, or sentence.

> The Phrase Completion Method is more complex than the *Embedded Question*, *Tell Me Phrase*, or *Alternate Choice*. If there is difficulty with recall or the PCD is not coming up with the word you are stimulating, you will want to use this method at a later time and just use the *Embedded Question*, *Tell Me Phrase*, or *Alternate Choice Questions*. You may need to work with some PCDs for months on the *Embedded Questions* and *Tell Me Phrases*. That is okay.
>
> There have been many PCDs with whom I could only do *Embedded Questions* and *Tell Me Phrases* for long periods of time. Sometimes I wondered if they would ever be able to answer a question without cueing them with the words from those methods. There were times when I contemplated giving up, and they would start coming around and answer a single *Embedded Question* without the *Tell Me Phrase*. If I asked them an open-ended question, they would finally answer the question with the right word all by themselves — a breakthrough!
>
> Never fret about how long you may have to use any given method. Just persist, and in time, you should get the results toward which you are working. What I am really saying here is that if your PCD does need the *Embedded Question* and the *Tell Me Phrases* month after month, do not worry. Stay with it, no matter how long it takes!

Example

SM: How about some hot _____? (coffee)

SM: Or maybe you want a small glass of _____? (juice, water, milk, etc.)

SM: I know what you like in your coffee; you like _____. (milk, cream, sugar, sweetener, Sweet & Low)

SM: How about a couple of scrambled _____? (eggs)

Just remember that we are only at a *Single-Word Level* in the above examples. It is relatively simple to shift from the *Single-Word Level* of language stimulation to two or three words, although for the new SM, I suggest that you employ the above strategies until both you and the PCD are proficient with them. Then go on to expanding the number of words in the utterances. Always stimulate words while looking at one another, as previously discussed in the initial section on mirroring. While you are stimulating speech, they will be looking at your lips, tongue, and mouth for cues to help them say the word.

How will you know when to begin stimulating utterances of more than one word? Simple. It is when the PCD can readily say single words in response to *Embedded Questions, Alternate Choice, What It Is?©* questions, or *Phrase Completion* statements without difficulty. You will know when they can do any one or all of the above. Before going on to the stimulation of phrases, I want you to remember that if a *Phrase Completion* exercise does not work, you can just work backwards to the *Embedded Question* or *Alternate Choice*. When you find a method that works, stay with it for a while and just have fun stimulating speech. Remember, there is no fire to put out. Take your time, talk about lots of cool stuff, and *embed* the answers into the question. In time, you should no longer have to do that.

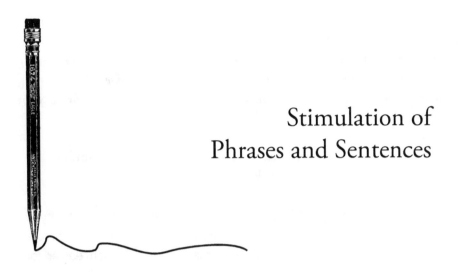

Stimulation of Phrases and Sentences

Combining Words into Sentences

We are now ready to progress to a *two-word language formulation* model. I typically do not spend a lot of time at the *Single-Word Level* unless the PCD has a severe apraxia or extreme difficulty imitating vowels or simple words. Other concerns that may be present deal with immediate memory and the necessity to keep stimulating single words over and over again, because there is minimal independent recall. You must remember that each person you stimulate is different. You must persist, even with those PCDs who do not always show immediate progress. I cannot tell you how many times I have been ready to give up when, as if by magic, they began to utter single words or word pairs with no cues or *Embedded Questions*.

I will move on to a *Two-Word Level* once the PCD shows improvement in readily comprehending my questions and answering/repeating the target word with immediate memory. The number of *Embedded Questions* and repetitions of *Tell Me Phrases* begins to diminish at this level. Once they are able to say single words, I want them to expand those *Single-Word Utterances* to a *Two-* or *Three-Word Level*. Remember that speech is a combination of subjects and predicates, or nouns and verbs. In the strategies for single words, I showed you a number of methods to stimulate talking using nouns, verbs, or adjectives. Those same techniques would also be beneficial when expanding or lengthening the response from the *Single-Word Response*. The following strategies and methods are designed to help you develop your proficiency for *Two-* and *Three-Word Responses*.

Embedded Questions with Tell Me Phrase for Short Two-Word or Three-Word Responses for I → Verb

 At this point, think of some *Two-Word Responses* that you would like the PCD to say, and write them down before proceeding with this exercise. It will be much easier for you to do this if you have taken some time to think of some simple *Two-Word Responses* or requests/answers that you would like to have them say.

When you stimulate, be as gestural and animated as you possibly can. Work on these combinations very slowly. You may want to take your hand and place it on your chest, open your mouth wide, and emphasize the word "I," which often is the subject of the sentence.

Example
SM:	Do you eat?
PCD:	(Nodding of the head)
SM:	YES?
PCD:	YES.
SM:	Tell me: I EAT.
PCD:	I EAT.

Place your hand on your chest; open your mouth wide, and give lots of visual and auditory cues for "I." Then complete the sentence slowly with the word "eat." Remember that you want the PCD to be an exact mirror of your mouth, jaw, and tongue movements. Therefore, say "I" and have them imitate "I." Then say "eat." You have now said "I" and they have said "I"; then you said "eat" and they said "eat." Soon, you will find yourselves saying phrases at the same time or in unison.

Additional Practice

Do you drink?

Do you watch? (TV)

Do you sit?

Do you stand?

Do you walk?

Do you pee?

Do you shower?

Do you bathe?

Do you brush hair?

Do you brush teeth?

Do you shave?

Do you comb? (hair)

Do you dress?

Do you write?

Do you read?

Do you go? (bank)

Do you go? (doctor)

Remember that in this strategy, we use the question. It can be confusing for the PCD when you say "Do you ➔ eat or drink." In the early stages of stimulation, the PCD may actually repeat the question or say "you eat" or "you drink." That is not what we want.

To assure correct responses, I emphasize in the next step, the *Tell Me Phrase* "I EAT."

Example

SM: Do you eat?

PCD: Uh hum.

SM: YES?

PCD: YES.

SM: Tell me: I ➔ verb ("I EAT") using "I."

Then put your hand on your chest and cue the word "I." Once you do this, say (the verb): "EAT." Now the PCD will utter: "I EAT" or "I WALK," or just about any combination of a noun or (subject ➔ verb).

Initially, simple *Two-Word Responses* such as "I eat," "I wash," or "I walk," etc., should be easily uttered by the PCD since you are conditioning them to say each word at the *Single-Word Level* with cues. Remember to stimulate each word with a clear and appropriately loud voice, and make sure to condition the word "I" with cues and gestures. It is a very important word for the PCD. Just practice with them to say the word "I," for it is one of the foundation blocks of the sentence, especially when you are dealing with someone who has a moderate to profound speech and language impairment. With training, in a very short time, all you will have to do is point to your chest and open your mouth for "I," and the PCD will be able to say that word and the verb readily.

Example

SM:	Do you EAT?
PCD:	(Nods and mmm)
SM:	YES?
PCD:	YES.
SM:	Tell me: I.
PCD:	I.
SM:	EAT.
PCD:	EAT.

Point to your chest and mouth or have the PCD mirror you when you say "I," followed by a gesture with your hand to your mouth to cue "eat." With a laptop or computer, type "I EAT" in large font separated with some space as another cue to stimulate the word pair after you ask the question, "Do you eat?" You could go on for days with questions about whether your PCD does a host of activities (verbs). Work on these utterances until it is a relatively simple task for the PCD.

Some PCDs will be at a more advanced level. They will be able to answer with more than a *One-Word Response*. In such cases, you would just ask a question, as in the following example:

SM:	Do you EAT?
PCD:	(Nods and mmmmmm)
SM:	YES?
PCD:	YES.

SM   Tell me: I EAT.
PCD: I EAT.

Later on, but probably not now, you should practice *Two-Word Responses* with the other methods presented thus far, such as the *Alternate Choice, Phrase Completion* and *What It Is?*© method.

Stimulating the I Want ➜ (Object) Sentence

Method: Stimulating a "Yes" Response
If the PCD is progressing nicely, you might be able to go to the next expansion of the utterance, which is the *I Want* ➜ (object) phrase.

SM: Do you want ➜ (Noun)?

It is very important here to make sure that you get an answer to your question. Do not proceed with the stimulation of the sentence until you receive a clear, nonverbal indication from the PCD using a calibrated "yes" or "no" and a verbal reply of "yes" or "no" using spoken words.

PCD: YES.

If they want what you are asking them, proceed to the *Tell Me Phrase.*

Tell me: I ➜ want ➜(Noun).

Point to your chest and begin the visual cue for "I," or show them the computer screen where you are typing: "I ➜ want ➜ (noun)." Since you know they can imitate, which is why you are at this level of language stimulation, you can see that your PCD is gaining a wealth of information about the sentence they are in the process of speaking:

Do you WANT LUNCH?

The PCD has heard the question with the verb and object in it.
The PCD has replied with a "YES" that was either spontaneously uttered without help, or cued with a *Tell Me Phrase.*

The PCD hears you say, "Tell me: I WANT LUNCH." ("Tell me" is spoken at a lower volume than "I WANT LUNCH," which is stated in an appreciably louder tone, conveying to the PCD that this is the phrase you want repeated.)

The PCD knows what to do when you gesture to your chest and open your mouth for the word "I" (to say it). He gets another visual cue from the gesture for "want," which is extending both of your arms out straight, pulling hands and arms in towards your chest, and saying the word "WANT" at the same time. You could also have typed on the computer screen, "I WANT LUNCH" (preferable, but not necessary, as long as they have some recognition and immediate memory of the simple words you are giving them). Typing it on the computer screen may also be good for reinforcing printed word recognition. There will of course be times when a computer is not accessible.

Next, you want them to say the phrase. You can, while facing the PCD, begin to say each word of the sentence with gestures and visual cues, and have them mirror you with simultaneous movement and speaking.

PCD: I WANT LUNCH.

The above examples are good when you are first training your PCD, and are generally used with people who are difficult to stimulate. You will find some who will respond perfectly to a simple question with training, such as:

Example
SM: Do you want milk?
PCD: (Nodding)
SM: YES?
PCD: YES.
SM: Tell me: I WANT MILK.
PCD: I WANT MILK.

If the subject can answer the question in one step, you can now ask them throughout the day: "Do you want _____?" In this way, speech can be generated by the SM all day long in the context of the PCD's home environment.

Example
SM: Do you want lunch?
PCD: (Nods head)

SM: YES?
PCD: YES.
SM: Tell me: I WANT LUNCH.
PCD: I WANT LUNCH.

What to do if the PCD does **NOT WANT** what you are asking.

Method: Stimulating a "No" Response

This is an interesting verbal interaction. There are many ways we can say "no" to a question, and we all do it every day.

Let's ponder for a moment what we would say if someone came up to us and asked if we wanted something. We could say: "No," "No thanks," "No thank you," or "I don't want ➔ (noun/object.)"

If you want to teach these responses to a person with a communication difficulty, it would be relatively simple providing you have followed the steps that I have presented thus far.

Example

SM: Do you want milk?
PCD: (Inaudible, but uses body language that indicates "no")
SM: Tell me: NO! (You may also type this out on your computer screen or write it in very large letters.)
PCD: NO. (The PCD should readily be saying "no" at this point.)

SM: Do you want milk?
PCD: (Inaudible, but uses body language that indicates "no")
SM: NO?
PCD: NO.
SM: Tell me: NO, THANKS! (You may also type this out on your computer screen or write it in very large letters.)

The PCD will either say "No, thanks" due to the conditioning they have received from you, or you may have to proceed with the next step.

The manual sign for "no" may vary from person to person. Some individuals finger-spell the word "no," and others use one, quick hand movement. The one I prefer is a flat, horizontal hand, palm facing the ground, beginning at the side of the SM's neck and swinging at arm's length and at neck height 180 degrees to the other side of the body. Now, give the manual sign for "no" and time the movement of your arm to be simultaneous with saying the words "NO ➔ THANKS." If they have articulation difficulties, make sure you place your tongue on the roof of your mouth in plain view for them, wait until they put their tongue on the roof of their mouth, and then you say "NNNNNNNNNNNNNNN (elongating the N), and then gliding that into a rounded mouth for the O: "Nnnnnnnnnnnoooooooooooooooooo." Next, proceed to "thanks," protruding your tongue between the upper and lower teeth or gums for the (th), making sure they do the same. Slowly glide and complete the word "THHHHHH---ANKS."

Repeat the above procedures for "No," "No thanks," "No, thank you."

Method : Stimulating Negative + Noun (Two-Word Responses)
Example (Two-Word Responses)

SM:	Do you want coffee?
PCD:	(Shakes head for "no")
SM:	No?
PCD:	(Shakes head for "no")
SM:	NO?
SM:	NO.
SM:	Tell me: NO COFFEE!
PCD:	NO COFFEE!
SM:	Maybe later? (Exploring the possibility for coffee later)
PCD:	NO.
SM:	Not later?
PCD:	NO.
SM:	Tell me: NOT LATER!
PCD:	NOT LATER!

Method: Stimulating I Don't Want Answers (Three- and Four-Word Responses)
Example (Three-Word)

SM:	Do you want cereal?
PCD:	(Shakes head for "no")
SM:	NO?
PCD:	NO.

SM: Tell me: I DON'T WANT (Say each word, one at a time: I →DON'T → WANT!)

PCD: I DON'T WANT!

SM: Do you want cereal?
PCD: (Shakes head for "no")
SM: NO?
PCD: NO.
SM: Tell me: NO, THANK YOU.
PCD: NO, THANKS.
SM: Tell me: NO, THANK *YOU*! (You are expanding the utterance by one word)
PCD: NO, THANK YOU.

SM: Do you want coffee?
PCD: (Shakes his head)
SM: NO?
PCD: NO.
SM: Tell Me: I DON'T WANT COFFEE. (I → DON'T → WANT → COFFEE)
SM: You ready? Say: I DON'T WANT COFFEE.
PCD: I DON'T WANT COFFEE.

You can then go through a host of questions that could be used when asking the PCD what they want or don't want during any ADL activity.

Method: Stimulating Alternate Choice Responses

> If the PCD easily responds to your *Alternate Choice Question* with a single word, begin stimulating a short sentence. Begin that process with a *Tell Me Phrase*, as in the example below.

Example

SM: Do you want cereal or eggs?
PCD: EGGS.

SM: Good. Tell me: I WANT EGGS.

PCD: I WANT EGGS.

SM: One or two eggs?

PCD: TWO EGGS.

SM: Good. Tell me: I WANT TWO EGGS!

PCD: I WANT TWO EGGS.

> Make sure that the PCD first answers easily with a single word, and then use a *Tell Me Phrase* to stimulate a short sentence. Please remember to give two choices.

Practice Time

Now practice the following examples by first getting a *One- to Four-Word Response* using the *Alternate Choice Model* reviewed thus far.

SM: Do you want WATER/JUICE?

SM: Do you want COFFEE/TEA?

SM: Do you want EGGS?

SM: Do you want FRIED/POACHED?

SM: Do you want BOILED/FRIED?

SM: Do you want ONE or TWO?

SM: Do you want CEREAL?

SM: Do you want HOT/COLD?

Method: Two-Word Responses of Verb → Object (Daily Routine)

We do many things throughout the day. This exercise deals with everything we might do on a daily basis. My request to you, the SM, is to practice stimulating everything that the PCD does each day in the context of the situation. So, if the PCD is getting dressed, stimulate "I dress." If they are eating, stimulate "I eat"; and so on.

 I will start this list for you, and then I want you to observe your PCD. *List everything they do, and write it in a notebook or type it into your word processor*. If I were to write everything a friend of mine does on a daily basis, it would include:

Example

Get up Do you want to get up? (if affirmative) Tell me: GET UP!

Go pee. Do you want to go pee? (if affirmative) Tell me: GO PEE!

Read the following list, starting at the left column and reading down.

◯	◯	
brush teeth	tie shoe	make bed
floss teeth	drink coffee	take bath
take shower	get computer	take shower
get in	plug in	get in
turn on	unplug computer	get out
wash hair	in bag	wash hair
wash body	straighten office to do list	brush teeth
shave face	get ready	dry off
turn off (water)	go work	open window
get out (shower)	go car	close window
grab towel	get in	too cold
dry off	key in	too hot
powder on	belt on	AC on
deodorant on	turn key	heat on
get underwear	start car	get coke
put on	let's go	get juice
get shirt	right now	no way
put on	not later	fix it
get pants	let's eat	want more
put on	right now	want it
get socks	get dressed	don't want
put on	go bathroom	go away
right shoe	go out	come here
put on	go doctor	water yard
left shoe	get mail	clean bathroom
put on	more coffee	make bed

The list can go on and on! Remember that you, the SM, must know in your head whether you are going to stimulate a *One-, Two-, Three-, or Four-Word Response*; and you must configure in your head <u>both</u> what you want the PCD to say and how you will ask the question to get the number of words you want before you engage them.

This list encompasses only a small fraction of what a person does on a daily basis. Your goal is to realize the rich opportunities you have to stimulate speech and language throughout the day, and to make sure you start at a point that is easy. Remember to be consistent and, if a PCD is at a *Single-Word Level*, only stimulate single-word responses until the PCD utters single words without difficulty – as if both of you could do it blindfolded. From there, go to the *Two-Word Response* and keep adding or expanding the length of utterances in word progressions until you achieve a proficiency at well over 95%. Then continue with *Three-* and *Four-Word Responses* on up, making sure that they can achieve a proficiency level of 95%+ before expanding and adding another word.

Method: Stimulating Two-Word Reponses with I → Verb

 I will get you started. Again, you may want to make a list of what your PCD does on a daily basis, and stimulate them as they go through the day. What is different about this exercise is the use of the pronoun "I" followed by the present tense verb. As the PCD continues through the day and while performing an activity, you could ask them:

Example

SM: Do you STAND?

PCD: STAND.

SM: Do you STAND?

PCD: (Nods head)

SM: YES?

PCD: YES.

SM: Tell Me: I STAND. (Always do your best to observe physiology for a "yes" or "no" before stimulating the phrase.)

PCD: I STAND.

◯			◯	
I stand	I sit	I pee	I wash	I shower
I wash	I go	I turn	I stop	I see
I dry	I get	I dress	I pick	I brush
I shave	I open	I close	I pet (dog)	I kiss
I walk	I talk	I read	I listen	I sit
I eat	I drink	I stand	I go	I walk
I sit	I watch (TV)	I change	I read	I stand
I pee	I poop	I laugh	I go	

You can go on and on with this exercise, and add more Subject → Verb combinations as you observe your PCD go through their day.

PCD Making Requests of You

Method: Stimulating Two-Word Responses With You → Verb

If you want the PCD to make requests, this is one possibility. Create a list similar to the one below of two-word requests that the PCD will be making of you.

Example

You help	Oh, you want me to help you?	Tell me: HELP ME	(Please)
You get	You want me to get something?	Tell me: GET_____	(Please)
You come	You want me to come?	Tell me: COME HERE	(Please)
You go	You want me to go away?	Tell me: GO AWAY	(Please)
You find	You want me to find_____?	Tell me: FIND _____	(Please)
You cook	You want me to cook_____?	Tell me: COOK _____	(Please)

Please list in a notebook or on a computer anything that your PCD may want or need from you so they can make the request.

The desire to speak is based on need, so please observe your PCD throughout the day. When they want or need something, that will be your golden opportunity to stimulate speech. Ask the *Embedded Question* and stimulate the response.

Method: Stimulating You → Verb, Please

(*Please* is a word that connotes courtesy and respect for the person to whom you are making requests.

Or, you can set it up for "you understood" requests (2 words).

Example

SM: You want me to (verb-object) _____? (See phrases below and add your own phrases to this list.)

help me	You want me to help you?	Tell me: HELP ME! (Please)
get cake	You want me to get cake?	Tell me: GET CAKE. (Please)
come here	You want me to come here?	Tell me: COME HERE. (Please)
go away	You want me to go away?	Tell me: GO AWAY! (Please)

○		○	
right now	get water	get soda
get cigarettes	get drinks	get food
find keys	cook dinner	make sandwich
make bed	do laundry	dry clothes
fold clothes	sweep floor	vacuum floor
wash dishes	put away	go walk
go doctor	cut grass	make steak
get chicken	get coke	take shower
get dressed	shave beard	get brush

Example

SM: You want me to (verb+object) _____?

 Please add phrases that are important for your PCD to your notebook or computer.

The I Am/Am Not Level of Language Formulation

Method: Embedded Question

Two- or *Three-Word Reponses* that describe how the PCD may be feeling. As you see below, you could stimulate this with either

I am _____, or

I'm _____.

The PCD who was once able to speak without difficulty may prefer to use the contraction "I'm_____" since we know that once language is learned and spoken, most people would rather use the contraction than the more formal "I am_____."

For the child or person who has never spoken, it may be more prudent to initially stimulate the formal use of "I am_____."

Practice asking the *Yes/No Question* with the *Tell Me Phrase*, or you could use the exercise of saying *What It Is©*.

Example

SM: Are you hot?

PCD: Mmmm.

SM: YES?

PCD: YES.

SM: Tell me: I AM HOT.

PCD: I AM HOT.

Use the *Tell Me Phrases* "*I'm/I am*" in the above *Embedded Question* models. If the PCD does not readily formulate the *Three-Word Response* after the question, "Are you _____?" then try the *What It Is©* method below.

Method: What It Is©

SM: I'm cold. Are you?

PCD: I'M COLD.

⬭		⬭
I'm cold	I'm thirsty	I'm hungry
I'm tired	I'm sleepy	I'm pissed
I'm happy	I'm angry	I'm depressed
I'm sick	I'm okay	I'm ready

Example

> SM: I'm hot. Are you?
> PCD: I'M HOT.
> SM: I'm cold. Are you?
> PCD: I'M COLD.

Method: What It Is with Negation

SM: I'm cold. Are you?
PCD: NO.
SM: You're not?
PCD: NO.
SM: Tell me: I'M NOT.
PCD: I'M NOT.

(Expanding to three words)

SM: Tell me: I'M NOT COLD!
PCD: I'M NOT COLD!

(Expanding to four words)

SM: Tell me: I AM NOT COLD!
PCD: I AM NOT COLD!

 In your notebook or on your computer, please list some of the feelings your PCD may experience on a regular basis. I will start you off with the examples below.

⭕			⭕	
angry	concerned	eager	grouchy	happy
hopeful	jealous	relaxed	sad	strong
bad	good	upset	weak	

The I Am Exercise

If your PCD is getting better at responding to the procedures for language stimulation covered so far, they might be able to do a fun little exercise.

This is called the *Am/Am Not Exercise*. It is fun. You can make the directions simple; similar to the ones with the *What It Is©* exercise.

The exercise for beginners *at the start of training* begins with the SM making a statement that is true and requiring the PCD to also make the statement. The SM knows ahead of time that the statement is true for the PCD also.-

 Create a list of things both of you ARE, using "am." Please do your best to create at least 25 statements –preferably more. You can use *predicate nouns, predicate adjectives,* or *progressive verbs (ing)*. Have fun with this and create interesting dialogue.

SM: I AM A MAN.   PCD: I AM A MAN.
SM: I AM A FATHER.   PCD: I AM A FATHER.
SM: I AM A HUSBAND.   PCD: I AM A HUSBAND.
SM: I AM RELAXED.   PCD: I AM RELAXED.
SM: I AM HERE.   PCD: I AM HERE.
SM: I AM HONEST.   PCD: I AM HONEST.
SM: I AM FRIENDLY.   PCD: I AM FRIENDLY.

Using the I Am ➔ (Verb+ing) to Describe Daily Activities

With these words in the I Am ➔ Verb-ing sequence, you can also have the PCD state what they are doing as the day unfolds in their *activities of daily living (ADLs)*. In this exercise, we are using the I Am ➔ (Verb-ing) to stimulate virtually hundreds of simple things the PCD may do on a daily basis following the above model.

You can also stimulate the present progressive tense in this exercise by first describing what you both are experiencing in the moment. Once you are able to do this, you can also stimulate small phrases by having the PCD tell you what they are doing in the moment throughout the day.

SM: I AM THINKING.	PCD: I AM THINKING.
SM: I AM TALKING.	PCD: I AM TALKING.
SM: I AM LISTENING.	PCD: I AM LISTENING.
SM: I AM SITTING.	PCD: I AM SITTING.
SM: I AM BREATHING.	PCD: I AM BREATHING.
SM: I AM SEEING.	PCD: I AM SEEING.
SM: I AM SMELLING.	PCD: I AM SMELLING.

Throughout the day, you can be asking:

SM: ARE YOU WAKING?	SM: ARE YOU SHOWERING?
SM: ARE YOU WALKING?	SM: ARE YOU DRYING?
SM: ARE YOU WASHING?	SM: ARE YOU SHAVING?
SM: ARE YOU DRESSING?	SM: ARE YOU COMBING?

 Now create a list in your notebook or computer regarding what you both ARE NOT. Please create a list of as many of these as you can; at least 25, and preferably more that will pertain to you and your person with the speaking difficulty. With training, you could do this exercise with or without printed words or photos. You can use predicate nouns, predicate adjectives, or progressive verbs (ing).

The I Am Not Exercise

SM: I AM NOT A WOMAN.	PCD: I AM NOT A WOMAN. (MAN)
SM: I AM NOT A MILLIONAIRE.	PCD: I AM NOT A MILLIONAIRE.
SM: I AM NOT COLD.	PCD: I AM NOT COLD.
SM: I AM NOT HUNGRY	PCD: I AM NOT HUNGRY.
SM: I AM NOT SINGING.	PCD: I AM NOT SINGING.
SM: I AM NOT WRITING.	PCD: I AM NOT WRITING.
SM: I AM NOT HOT.	PCD: I AM NOT HOT.

SM: I AM NOT THIRSTY.   PCD: I AM NOT THIRSTY.

SM: I AM NOT BAD.   PCD: I AM NOT BAD.

I Am Not Verb+ing

SM: I AM NOT READING.   PCD: I AM NOT READING.

SM: I AM NOT DANCING.   PCD: I AM NOT DANCING.

SM: I AM NOT SLEEPING.   PCD: I AM NOT SLEEPING.

SM: I AM NOT SNORING.   PCD: I A NOT SNORING.

Once the PCD can perform the above exercises with excellent accuracy (98% range), you can "change it up," and present negative (not) and positive (am) comments spontaneously from either category, and see if your PCD can supply the answer that applies to them. By now, you should know if they can accomplish this.

SM: I AM A FATHER.   PCD: I AM NOT A FATHER.

SM: I AM BAPTIST.   PCD: I AM NOT BAPTIST.

SM: I AM NOT GOING HOME.   PCD: I AM GOING HOME.

SM: I AM TIRED.   PCD: I AM NOT TIRED.

SM: I AM NOT TALKING.   PCD: I AM TALKING.

SM: I AM NOT LISTENING.   PCD: I AM LISTENING.

SM: I AM NOT BREATHING.   PCD: I AM BREATHING.

The person with the speaking difficulty should begin to *generate* speech after a while. By that, I mean that they will *begin supplying responses that are not expected.*

The other day I said to one PCD: "I am tired." He said: "I feel great" — totally different words than what I expected. From that point on, he started using more *independent language* (his own language), which was NOT modeled for him. What this shows is language at the *generative stage.* That occurs when the PCD starts to use his own vocabulary and expressions. Generative or independent language is the result of the language structures that have been practiced and modeled using the earlier, elementary levels of the *Embedded Question, Alternate Choice, Phrase Completion,* and *What It Is©* exercises. For the normal-speaking person, speech and the use of language are spontaneous, unexpected, and *reactive.* We *react* to what is said to us. These exercises, with time and practice, are designed to lead the PCD to react automatically to what is spoken or said to them at a generative level. This leads to more natural speaking ability; and, BINGO! That's what we want! The satisfaction of hearing and seeing our PCD generate speech independently is fabulous and reminds us of the true gift we have of helping people speak or speak again. It has always been the reason I get out of bed in the morning, and I hope it will be the same for you!

Remember, when you are working on these language responses, start with the approximate number of words the PCD is using comfortably at the time you begin working together. If the PCD speaks using single words only, start there and expand the number of words, one word at a time. If two or three words seem to be common when the PCD attempts to speak, begin all exercises in this book at the two-word level. If the person you are working with is speaking in four-word phrases, that is where you start and expand by one word when you reach a consistency of over 95%.

 List all the things that are requested in a typical day and make sure you are asking the *Yes/No Question* and embedding the target word in your question.

Practicing Requests (I Want)

I Do/Don't Want → Objects (Three-Word Responses)

Example

(Positive Response)

SM: Do you want coffee?

PCD: (Nods head "yes")

SM: YES?

PCD: YES.

SM: Tell me: I WANT → COFFEE.

PCD: I WANT → COFFEE.

(Negative Response)

SM: Do you want COFFEE?

PCD: (Shakes head "no")

SM: NO?

PCD: NO.

SM: Tell me: I DON'T → WANT COFFEE.

PCD: I DON'T → WANT COFFEE.

You can stimulate the phrases "I DON'T" and "WANT COFFEE" separately or you can combine them if your PCD is stimulable.

 Remember this is only a guide for the words you will choose. The way to add words to your lexicon (vocabulary list) is to be keenly aware of the things (words) and events that take place each day in the life of your PCD – the wants, needs, and requests; the frustrations as well as the successes – and add those words to your lists.

I Want ➔ *Verb (Three-Word Responses)*

Example

If you are still at a rather primary level of two or three words, you can stimulate requests with:

I WANT ➔ (VERB)

SM:	Do you want undress?
PCD:	(Nods)
SM:	YES?
PCD:	YES.
SM:	Tell me: I WANT UNDRESS.
PCD:	I WANT UNDRESS.

For those people who are doing well with this method, you may only be able to stimulate three words. However, if your PCD is at a more advanced level, or if these methods are too easy, you might stimulate the infinitive (to ➔ verb) instead of the above exercise, as shown below. The infinitive is explained following this strategy.

Example

I WANT TO ➔ VERB

SM:	Do you want to (verb) sleep?
PCD:	(Nods)
SM:	YES?
PCD:	YES.
SM:	Tell me: I WANT TO ➔ SLEEP (VERB).
PCD:	I WANT TO ➔ SLEEP (VERB).

I Want → Noun (Three-Word Responses)
I WANT → NOUN

SM: Do you want pills?
PCD: (Nods)
SM: YES?
PCD: YES.
SM: Tell me: I WANT → PILLS (NOUN).
PCD: I WANT → PILLS (NOUN).
SM: Tell me again: I WANT PILLS.
PCD: I WANT PILLS.

I Want → (Verb) (Object/Noun)
Example

SM: Do you want drink coke? or
SM: Do you want come outside?

Verbs	Nouns
drink	coke
eat	bagel
go	Wal-Mart
sweep	driveway
clean	bathroom
come	outside
wear	dress
undress	clothes
sleep	bed
call	mom
get	medicine
buy	soda
read	mail
see	children
smell	cookies
hear	music

feel	rain
clean	hands
ride	car
travel	someplace
talk	sister
listen	president
learn	talking
have	computer

 Please list in your notebook or on your computer as many verb ➜ noun requests as you can think of that the PCD may need to make.

I want eat dinner.
I want wash hands.
I want take shower.

Using the I ➜ (Verb) (Predicate) to Describe Daily Activities

With these words in the verb ➜ *predicate sequence*, you can then have the PCD state what they are doing as the day unfolds in their *activities of daily living (ADLs)*. In an earlier exercise, I had you stimulating simple I ➜ verb (page 70) or verb ➜ noun/object utterances (pages 79 and 107).

In this strategy, whatever the *activity* that the PCD is doing (within reason), you are **asking them the question** to get a full sentence in reply.

SM: Do you get up?	PCD: I GET UP.
SM: Do you go pee?	PCD: I GO PEE.
SM: Do you take shower?	PCD: I TAKE SHOWER.
SM: Do you get dressed?	PCD: I GET DRESSED.

You can stimulate virtually hundreds of simple things the PCD may do on a daily basis following the above model.

I Want (to ➔ Verb Infinitive)

Requests:

I want to go.	I want to eat.	I want to nap.
I want to buy.	I want to wash.	I want to shower.
I want to bathe.		

 In your notebook or on your computer, make a list of what your PCD wants on a daily basis.

List Nouns: (things, places, persons)
List Verbs: (to eat, to watch, to drink, etc.)

Example
Using the I Want (to ➔ Verb) (Object)

Do you want to eat ➔ CHICKEN?
Do you want to drink ➔ COKE?
Do you want to go ➔ BANK?
Do you want to take ➔ NAP?
Do you want to go ➔ OUT?

This method can be generative, i.e., you could then ask almost any question to get almost any utterance. To show you that concept, what follows is an example of a line of questioning.

Example
Third Person Progressive Tense Exercise

SM:	Suzie is coming over.
SM:	Is Suzie coming over?
PCD:	Yes.
SM:	Is Suzie coming over?
PCD:	Yes, Suzie.
SM:	Good. Tell me: SUZIE IS COMING OVER!
PCD:	SUZIE COMING OVER.
SM:	Good. Tell me: SUZIE **IS* COMING OVER**. (*Bold and enlarged type indicates how to emphasize words you want PCD to insert.)

PCD: SUZIE **IS** COMING OVER.

SM: Is Momma going to bed?
PCD: Yes.
SM: Tell me: MOMMA IS GOING TO BED.
PCD: MOMMA GOING BED.
SM: Tell me: MOMMA **IS GOING TO** BED!
PCD: MOMMA IS GOING TO BED.

If the PCD cannot get all of the words from the *Tell Me Phrase*, particularly if they are leaving out the **is** and **to**, emphasize them and slow down the *Tell Me Phrase*. If five words are just too many words, shorten the sentence by one or two words.

Four-word model rather than the above five-word model
Example
    SM: Is Momma in bed?
    PCD: Yes.
    SM: Tell me: MOMMA IS IN BED.
or
    SM: Momma went to bed? (Four-word *Embedded Question* model)
    PCD: Yes.
    PCD: Tell me: MOMMA WENT TO BED.
    PCD: MOMMA WENT TO BED.

Remember, you have a choice about HOW you want to go about stimulating language. You could stimulate it in the actual context of the situation, and you could stimulate speech and language in a workbook or picture book. *The Teaching of Talking* method is based on the premise that both can be helpful; however, one of the guiding principles of *The Teaching of Talking* is for the speech-language pathologist or caregiver or SM to get away from being tied to materials, books, or computers. By being free of them, you can stimulate speech all day long in whatever activity you are doing, and *keep the conversation interesting and relevant to the moment*. Not only that, but you can have the breakthrough of *dancing in the conversation* that we shall discuss later. This is the point at which the *doing* of the speech and language stimulation disappears and an honest to goodness conversation emerges, *time distortion* occurs, and the *time in conversation* goes by rapidly.

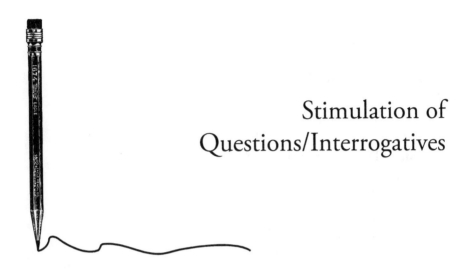

Stimulation of Questions/Interrogatives

Other Types of Questions (Interrogative) and How to Stimulate Them

You may be finding the stimulation of speech and language somewhat easier now. A question is very similar to stimulating a statement.

Typical everyday questions are as follows; however, please make sure you <u>pay very close attention</u> to your PCD and <u>note the questions they may ask.</u>

Who Is It/That?
Example
SM: Do you want to know, Who is it/that?

PCD: (Nods)

SM: YES?

PCD: YES.

SM: Ask me: WHO IS IT? or WHO IS THAT?

SM: Do you want to know WHO ARE THEY?

PCD: (Nods)

SM: YES?
PCD: YES.
SM: Ask me: WHO ARE THEY?
PCD: WHO ARE THEY?

What Are Those (Plural)?
Example
SM: Do you want to know, What are those?
PCD: (Nods)
SM: YES?
PCD: YES.
SM: Ask me: WHAT ARE THOSE?
PCD: WHAT ARE THOSE?

SM: Do you want to know, What is (the) time?
PCD: Mmmmmm.
SM: YES?
PCD: YES.
SM: Ask me: WHAT IS (THE) TIME?
PCD: WHAT IS TIME?

> Optional: With more advanced PCDs, you can add an extra word ("the") to extend the word count and make the sentence complete.

SM: Do you want to know what time it is?
PCD: Mmmmmm.
SM: YES?
PCD: YES.
SM: Ask me: WHAT TIME → IS IT?
PCD: WHAT TIME → IS IT?

When Is It/That?
Example
SM: Do you want to know, When is the show?
PCD: (Nods)
SM: YES?
PCD: YES.
SM: Ask me: WHEN IS (THE) SHOW?
PCD: WHEN IS SHOW?

When Are _____ (Plural)?
Example

SM: Do you want to know, When are we going?

PCD: (Nods)

SM: YES?

PCD: YES.

SM: Ask me: WHEN ARE → WE GOING?

PCD: WHEN ARE → WE GOING?

(These can be said in *Two-Word chunks*.)

Where Is It/That?
Where Are_____ (Plural)?
Example

SM: Do you want to know, Where are (the) keys?

PCD: (Nods)

SM: YES?

PCD: YES.

SM: Ask me: WHERE ARE (the) KEYS?

PCD: WHERE ARE KEYS?

How Is It/That?
Example

SM: You want to know, how is it?

PCD: (Nods)

SM: YES?

PCD: YES.

SM: Ask me: HOW IS IT/THAT?

PCD: HOW IS IT/THAT?

How Are _____ (You; Second Person or Third Person Plural)?
Example

SM: Do you want to know how I am?

PCD: (Nods)

SM: YES?

PCD: YES.

SM: Ask me: HOW ARE YOU?
PCD: HOW ARE YOU?

Stimulating the Who Is It/That Question

SM: Do you want to know who that is?
PCD: (Nods)
SM: YES?
PCD: YES.
SM: Can you ask: WHO IS ➜ IT/THAT?
PCD: WHO IS IT/THAT?
SM: Good. Can you tell me: WHO IS ➜ IT/THAT again?
PCD: WHO IS IT/THAT?

SM: Do you want to know who they are?
PCD: (Nods)
SM: YES?
PCD: YES.
SM: Excellent. Ask me: WHO ARE THEY?
PCD: WHO ARE THEY?

If you want to take it a step further to a statement, it could go something like this:

SM: Who is she?
SM: Tell me: WHO IS SHE?
PCD: WHO IS SHE?
SM: IS SHE JUDY?
PCD: Oh.
SM: Can you tell me: SHE IS JUDY.
PCD: JUDY.
SM: Can you tell me: SHE IS JUDY.
PCD: SHE IS JUDY.

Stimulating the What Is It Question

SM:Do you want to know what it is?
PCD: (Nodding)
SM: YES?

PCD: YES.

SM: Can you say: WHAT IS IT?

PCD: WHAT IS IT?

SM: Great.

SM: Can you ask me again: WHAT IS IT?

PCD: WHAT IS IT?

This is also a wonderful opportunity for the SM to stimulate a phrase from the PCD.

SM: IT'S AN ANT!

PCD: Mmmmmmm.

SM: Can you tell me: IT'S ➜ **AN** ➜ ANT!

PCD: ****IT IS ANT!****

**Note that PCD did not include "an" in his utterance. This utterance can be accepted for now, or the SM can test to see if he can get the complete utterance requested.

If the SM decides to see if he can get the complete utterance from the PCD, he would proceed as follows:

SM: I like the way you said IT IS ANT. Now we are going to add one more word to IT IS ANT. Can you say IT'S **AN** ANT?

PCD: IT'S AN ANT.

Stimulating Where Is/Are the _____ Questions

Years ago my children enjoyed a series of books called "Where's Waldo?" They had to find Waldo, who was hidden, along with dozens of other characters doing a variety of amusing things, across a two-page spread of pictures.

Many people who have strokes, aphasia, and brain injuries often misplace things and may need to ask where they are. The "*Where is_____?*" (noun/object) question is very common among those with speaking and cognitive difficulties. Come to think of it, wives may consider "*Where is _____*" to be the most frequently asked question of husbands and children, as well!

With this exercise, you can stimulate two different aspects: first, the inquiry of *where* something is, and second, lengthening the utterance to include prepositions, which state *where* something is. Here are some of the basic prepositions: in, on, under, around, above, below, and so on. Listed below are some of the common questions asked when wanting to know *where something is*.

> *Where is/are (the)* _____?

Review

If you want to stimulate the PCD to ask "where is" questions:

SM: You want to ask me: Where is the cat?
PCD: Mmmmmm.
SM: YES?
PCD: YES.
SM: Just ask me: WHERE IS (THE) CAT?
PCD: CAT.
SM: Good. Ask me: WHERE IS (THE) CAT?
PCD: WHERE IS CAT?
SM: Good. Ask me again: WHERE IS (THE) CAT?
PCD: WHERE IS CAT?

SM: You want to ask me: Where are the keys?
PCD: Mmmmmm.
SM: YES?
PCD: YES.
SM: Just ask me: WHERE ARE (THE) KEYS?
PCD: KEYS.
SM: Good. Ask me: WHERE ARE (THE) KEYS?
PCD: WHERE ARE KEYS?
SM: Good. Ask me again. WHERE ARE (THE) KEYS?
PCD: WHERE ARE KEYS?

Therefore, in the future, when the PCD wants to know *where* something is, you stimulate them with the above type of format.

> *Where is/are (the)* _____? (use of "the" is optional)

◯			◯	
Remote	key/keys	dog	dog food	my money
pen, pencil	paper	the phone	the bill	the mail
the book	the car	the shoes	the pants	the shirts
the cookies	the candy (etc.)			

If the PCD wants to know where something is and is unable to state the question, you can say something like this:

SM: You want to know, Where are keys?

PCD: Mmmmmm.

SM: YES?

PCD: YES.

SM: So ask me: WHERE ARE KEYS?

PCD: KEYS?

SM: Good. Ask me: WHERE ➜ ARE ➜ KEYS?"

SM: Tell me: WHERE ARE KEYS?

PCD: WHERE ARE KEYS?

At this point you can type out on your computer "Where are keys?" or you can just use the *Tell Me Phrase* with the question, as stated above.

PCD: WHERE ARE KEYS?

SM: Good. Tell me again: WHERE ARE KEYS?

PCD: WHERE ARE KEYS?

Locatives: Identifying Statements with Prepositions

You can now stimulate the statement of where the keys are, if your PC can say words in longer phrases. If he can say one word, you stimulate that; if he can say three or four, then you can stimulate a short statement such as:

SM: THE KEYS ARE IN KITCHEN.

PCD: KITCHEN.

SM: Can you say: KEYS ARE IN KITCHEN?

PCD: KEYS ARE IN KITCHEN.

In the above example, not only did we stimulate the question "Where are_____?" but we also stimulated the answer that is now expanded to: The (subject)_____are (preposition) the _____(object/predicate noun).

Example
The keys are <u>in</u> (the) kitchen. / The keys are <u>on</u> (the) table.

When the PCD Asks if YOU Want Something

Do you want (a/an)_____? (noun)
Or Do you want (to) _____ (verb)?

Or expanded to: DO YOU WANT TO VERB → NOUN OR OBJECT?

◯			◯	
go	eat	drink	sit	yell
cry	watch	shower	clean	drive
travel	leave	coke	bagel	steak
dinner				

SM:	Do you want to ask me if I want to go?
PCD:	(Nods)
SM:	YES?
PCD:	YES.
SM:	Ask me: DO YOU WANT TO GO?
PCD:	YOU GO?
SM:	Good. Ask me: DO YOU → WANT TO → GO? (chunked into two-word combinations)
or	
SM:	Good. Ask me: DO YOU → WANT TO → GO NOW? (chunked into 3 two-word combinations)

Notice that chunking into *Two-* or *Three-Word Responses* might be easier for the PCD to recall from immediate memory than the original question of five words: "DO YOU WANT TO GO?"

This could be a what, when, where, or how question; or, the PCD might be asking one of the following:

Example
What is that?
When are we going?
When is dinner?
Do you want _____?
Do you want to (go, eat, drink, sit, yell, get, visit, clean, drive, leave, help me, etc. — I think you get the picture...)

Example

SM:	Sometimes you want to know if I AM READY, right?
PCD:	(Nods head)
SM:	YES?
PCD:	YES.
SM:	So here we go. Ask if I am ready. Ask me: ARE YOU READY?
PCD:	Mmmmmm.
SM:	YES?
PCD:	YES.
SM:	So you want to ask me if I am ready?
PCD:	(Nodding)
SM:	YES?
PCD:	YES.
SM:	Ask me: ARE YOU READY?
PCD:	ARE YOU READY?
SM:	Yes. Very good.
SM:	Ask me again: ARE YOU READY?
PCD:	ARE YOU READY?
SM:	Ask me again: ARE YOU READY?
PCD:	ARE YOU READY?

Expanding the Length of the Question
The SM can also expand that question to more words with more advanced PCDs:

SM:	Would you like to ask me if I am ready to go?
PCD:	(Nods)

SM: YES?

PCD: YES.

SM: Ask me: ARE YOU READY TO GO?

PCD: (Nodding)

SM: YES?

PCD: YES.

SM: Ask Me: ARE YOU READY ➔ TO GO?

PCD: Mmmmm.

PCD: (Nods)

SM: YES?

PCD: YES.

SM: Ask me: ARE YOU READY ➔ TO GO?

PCD: ARE YOU READY ➔ TO GO?

For the more advanced PCD, you may work up to the following question:

SM: Do you want to know if I am READY TO GO?

PCD: Mmmmmm.

SM: YES?

PCD: YES.

SM: Ask me: ARE YOU READY ➔ TO GO?

PCD: ARE YOU READY ➔ TO GO?

SM: Want to ask me: ARE YOU READY ➔ TO GO TO ➔ THE MOVIES?

PCD: ARE YOU READY GO MOVIES?

    This is a good response and perfectly acceptable if you have been slowly rebuilding phrases and sentences. Be careful about expanding with too many words. The PCD will always let you know by what they say in response to your question whether the question you are providing is of adequate or excessive length.

Now, try to expand the following response from the PCD:

PCD: ARE YOU READY GO MOVIES?

SM: Good. Let's make it longer. Would that be okay with you?

PCD: Okay.

SM: Ask Me: ARE YOU READY → TO GO TO → MOVIES? (TO GO TO: set off with slower speed and emphasize each word.) (You can also help the PCD with three-word chunking, which is easier than trying to remember seven words.)

PCD: ARE YOU READY → **TO GO TO** → MOVIES?

Review

1. Stimulating language often requires a question.
2. Make sure you calibrate their "*Yes/No*" and then stimulate them to say "*Yes*" or "*No,*" so that you will know how to ask the next question which will lead to their verbal response.
3. Think of the utterance you want the PCD to learn and say.
4. Whether it is a one-, two-, four-, or six-word utterance, *construct a question of appropriate length to the answer you want. It* will have the *answer embedded* within it. Say the *Tell Me Phrase* with urgency, so that you can give the PCD the words of the utterance a second time. (The words for the utterance are therefore embedded within the question and the *Tell Me Phrase.*)
5. Use this technique so you can stimulate the PCD to *make statements* or *ask questions at any time or place.*

After a while you can use this method conversationally, and the PCD will not even consciously know what you are doing. You can learn how to *start the PCD off with consistent utterances of single words,* as long as you are *consistently asking questions and Tell Me Phrases for single words.* Then increase the number of words that the PCD is saying by consistently asking questions which are longer in nature, and using *Tell Me Phrases* or verbiage that is tolerated and will elicit the longer utterances.

Example

SM: Do you want to go over to Bob's house this afternoon?

To your surprise, the PCD may say:

PCD: Yeah, I want to go over to Bob's this afternoon.

SM: You want to take a cake with us?

PCD: Yes, let's take a cake.

I am including an actual conversation that took place with a PCD so you can see the beauty of the procedure and how simple it is. You will not need the *Tell Me Phrase* once you begin conditioning the PCD. They will start to automatically utter the language needed for the answer from your question, if you posed it properly and consistently.

Home Program	
Are you married?	Yes, I am married.
Are you a father?	Yes, I am a father.
Are you a son?	Yes, I am a son.
Are you a brother?	Yes, I am a brother.
Are you talking?	Yes, I am talking.
Are you on time?	Yes, I am on time.
Do you stretch your arm?	Yes, I stretch my arm.
Do you sit up straight?	Yes, I sit up straight.
Are you listening?	Yes, I am listening.
Are you speaking better?	Yes, I am speaking.
Are you awake?	Yes, I am awake.
Are you thin?	Yes, I am thin.
Are you strong?	Yes, I am strong.
Are you sitting down?	Yes, I am sitting down.
Are you thinking?	Yes, I am thinking.
Is she young?	Yes, she is young.
Is she pretty?	Yes, she is pretty.
Is she smiling?	Yes, she is smiling.
Is she listening?	Yes, she is listening.
Are you not a good boy?	No, I am not a good boy.
Are you patient?	Yes, I am patient.
Is she doing well?	Yes, she is doing well.
Is she talking?	Yes, she is talking.
Is she a student?	Yes, she is a student.
Is she helping us?	Yes, she is helping us.
Is she patient?	Yes, she is patient.
Is she kind?	Yes, she is kind.

A person I have been treating for a profound speaking difficulty follows a procedure each morning that goes something like the example below. Imagine — you could be doing something like this with your loved one or PCD!

SM	PCD
Are you ready to get up?	I'M READY. (Or: I'M READY TO GET UP.)
Are you going to pee?	I'M GOING TO PEE.
Do you want your walker?	I WANT MY WALKER.
Are you ready for a shower?	I'M READY. (Or: I'M READY FOR SHOWER.)
Will you brush your teeth?	I WILL BRUSH MY TEETH.
Will you shave now?	I WILL SHAVE NOW.
Will you wash hair?	I WILL WASH HAIR.
Are you finished?	
Say: I AM FINISHED.	I AM FINISHED. (Or: I'M FINISHED.)
Will you dry off?	I WILL DRY OFF.
Do you want the towel?	I WANT THE TOWEL.
Are you drying?	
Tell Me: I AM DRYING.	I AM DRYING.
Are you dry?	I AM DRY.
Do you want to dress?	I WANT TO DRESS.
Do you want briefs or boxers?	I WANT BRIEFS. (*Alternate Choice* method)
Blue socks or black socks?	BLACK SOCKS (*Alternate Choice*)
Do you want the white shirt?	I WANT WHITE SHIRT.
Do you want lunch now?	I WANT LUNCH NOW.
Do you want pizza or Chinese food?	CHINESE FOOD (*Alternate Choice*)

You will not always need to require a sentence response, although the stimulation of sentences is crucial to redeveloping the ability to talk, since we all speak in continuous speech and short utterances.

Look at the example above: "Do you want pizza or Chinese food?" If the PCD occasionally answers in a two-word utterance, such as "Chinese food," realize that many of us answer in short phrases when given a choice. However, when possible go for the "gold" and get the full sentence.

This type of questioning can go on all day long in the context of daily living. When the PCD is given questions that are of appropriate length and difficulty, his ability to listen and his immediate memory improves. He or she can readily answer a question with the correct structure since the PCD has been listening for the sounds, speed, grammar and syntax embedded within each question.

An interesting phenomenon will likely occur as the weeks and months progress. That is, the PCD will begin to respond with their own verbiage to questions and comments. They may, as if by magic, stop responding with the grammar and words that they heard within the question or statement and will begin to answer or *respond with a language all their own* —what I have coined *"independent language."* This is what I refer to as the *Prognostic Moment*. At this moment, and most probably in the future, this phenomenon will continue to occur until the PCD is conversing with his own language, filled with the richness of individualized *verbal mannerisms* and expressions of speech.

"I'll Tell You about Me, if You Tell Me about You"

Remember that it is all about modeling. That is, the PCD will be getting the "gold" of their speaking (the sounds, clarity, speed, grammar, syntax, morphology, etc.) that is embedded in your statement or question. They can also benefit from what you print on the legal pad or word processor/computer screen while you are speaking since it will reinforce the desired words, length and order of what will be spoken.

I have just finished reading an excellent book that is on the bestseller list, "Moonwalking with Einstein: The Art and Science of Remembering Everything," by Joshua Foer. In this most interesting book, Foer writes about people who are able to remember vast amounts of information by using mental imagery, and attaching what one wants to remember to a visual image of something or someplace familiar in the individual's experience. With this in mind, the following exercise is helpful for the PCD who is saying phrases and sentences through stimulation with any of the previous methods discussed.

I personally like this exercise, since it allows the PCD to generate some answers that are not given in the modeled question or *Tell Me Phrase*. In a way, the PCD has a task that is similar to the *Phrase Completion Method*, but the *I'll*

Tell You about Me, If You Tell Me about You Method is different. I will now give you the transcript of what a session might look like when you and the PCD are at a more advanced level of interaction.

Example

SM: Hi, John. We are going to have a conversation. I am going to share some of the things I know about me, and I am going to ask you to share some of the things you know about you.

So, I will tell you something about me. If it is the same for you, you say what I say. If I tell you something about me, and it is different for you, I want you to say a sentence and change what I say to make it right for you.

SM: I am a man; how about you?

PCD: I AM A MAN.

SM: I am ____ (age); how about you?

PCD: I AM 51.

SM: I am married. How about you?

PCD: I AM SINGLE.

SM: I am a speech pathologist. How about you?

PCD: I AM A CHEMIST.

SM: I am a bike rider. How about you?

PCD: I AM NOT A BIKE RIDER.

SM: I am from New Jersey. How about you?

PCD: I AM FROM NEW MEXICO.

SM: I am an American. How about you?

PCD: I AM AN AMERICAN.

SM: I am a homeowner. How about you?

PCD: I AM A HOMEOWNER.

SM: I am a gardener. How about you?

PCD: I'M NOT A GARDENER.

SM: I am a Democrat/Republican. How about you?

PCD: I'M A REPUBLICAN.

SM: I am a college grad. How about you?

PCD: I AM A COLLEGE GRAD.

SM: I have four kids. How about you?

PCD: I HAVE TWO KIDS.

SM: I have one daughter. How about you?

PCD: I HAVE NO DAUGHTERS.

SM: I have three sons. How about you?

PCD: I HAVE TWO SONS.

SM: I have a Toyota. How about you?

PCD: I HAVE A FORD.

SM: I have three bedrooms. How about you?

PCD: I HAVE THREE BEDROOMS.

SM: I have a dog. How about you?

PCD: I DON'T HAVE DOG.

SM: I like TV. How about you?

PCD: I LIKE TV.

SM: I like movies. How about you?

PCD: I LIKE MOVIES.

In this strategy, the simple sentence is given in the first part of my statement, and is followed by "How about you?" I will usually introduce at least ten of these "I have a _____. How about you?" statements. I will tell them I have a home, a dog, a Toyota, a daughter, etc., using the same structure each and every time. We change to a different statement when we get tired of telling each other what we have; we might then share what we like instead. "I like motorcycles. How about you?" We can share foods and beverages we enjoy, places we like, or people we know. When the target sentence of the exercise is kept consistent such as "I have," or "I like_____," it is easier for the PCD to reply. All he or she really has to think about is the answer, and if the statement and answer are easy enough, the response in the form of a phrase or sentence will be easy.

This strategy can also go on and on within a conversation for an hour or more. You can talk about anything from the music you like to the food, restaurants, TV shows, or sports you enjoy. And it's great, because the two of you are talking about what turns you on and finding your similarities and differences. After all, that's what conversations are for: to find our differences and similarities while speaking with one another. Once you find areas of similarities, you can speak more deeply on that subject, by remembering to make a simple statement followed by, "How about you?"

The other day I was doing therapy with someone who was from New York. I said:

SM: I'm from New Jersey; how about you?

PCD: I'M FROM NEW YORK.
SM: Cool. I love the Yankees.
PCD: YEAH, I LOVE THE METS!

Within a few minutes we were talking about the Yankees and the Mets and Yankee Stadium and Shea Stadium and Mickey Mantle and Roger Maris. Soon, we were conversing automatically. The fact that he had a severe speech problem disappeared, and I was deeply engaging him in conversation! He forgot that he had a problem and so did I. We were just caught up in the conversation that started out with a "therapy technique," and were so "into" the conversation that we ended up dancing in the conversation, which means that one gets caught up in a conversation and loses track of time, and that time actually *distorts*. When I say "distort," I'm referring to the idea that time passes *in the blink of an eye*. Have you ever been so engaged in a conversation that you looked down at your watch and could not believe that two or more hours had passed?

What you want to remember about this wonderful technique is to start out with lots of "I am's," then "I have's," then "I like's," or "I don't like's." Before you know it, the conversation will take on a life of its own. The two of you will be conversing with one another, and the "awareness" of the speaking difficulty will seemingly disappear, since you are now in what I have coined the "*communication sphere of consciousness*." Here, it really does not matter what or how something is being said, but rather that the two of you are expressing yourselves in whatever way works, and that the conversation has life and purpose. Most of all, there is information being conveyed, one to another.

For the person who has been seemingly unable to speak, an experience like this is a breakthrough for him or her, and for all concerned. When you get to this landmark of the *communication sphere of consciousness* within a conversation, you may want to stop expanding, correcting, etc., and just be present,[17] allowing the PCD to express themselves without having to do any therapy. Just have fun and converse. Allow whatever language is expressed, without any interruption.

This is the point at which the level of *independent language* emerges, the prognostic moment in which you both become aware that the conversation took off *on its own,* and that the PCD was talking *on their own*. It reminds me of the time I was teaching my son to ride a bike. I was running with him, my hand

---

17   Sims Wyeth & Co., "Communication Skills: Presence in Conversation," High Stakes Presentations, accessed September 25, 2009. http://www.simswyeth.com/20090925-communication-skills-presence-in-conversation/.

firmly on the seat. I finally let go, and there he was, riding down the road by himself —until he realized it, and then he fell down!

When the PCD starts to use independent language with the use of *The Teaching of Talking* method, allow for spontaneous conversation. For the person who has been unable to talk or speak for months, this will be a time of great exuberance. Just let him say whatever he wants, in whatever way he wishes to say it, and you will begin to see the sentence length, grammar, and complexity change on its own. Allow him the time to express himself, and do not interrupt unless you find that he is "stuck." If that happens, you can ask an *Embedded Question* pertaining to what he was talking about to get him on track, or recreate a conversation, which we shall get to shortly. Many PCDs will want to come in and just "talk," and not do any formal "stimulated work." Remember, for those of you who are less flexible, let them talk and be fully self-expressed. Let the river of conversation flow in the direction that it wants. At this point, you can take a more passive role in therapy by just asking them interesting questions about themselves, such as autobiographical facts; or, the two of you could take turns and just let each other know something interesting about yourselves. Often, by allowing the PCD to speak and express themselves, the grammar and syntax start to reemerge on their own. If they don't, you can help with the methods you have learned. However, let the person who is now speaking enjoy that privilege for a while without correcting, expanding, or clarifying unless completely necessary. In other words, imagine that the PCD has been locked up in "the speech jail," and is now being let out! Allow them to test out their new independence.

Recreating a Conversation

There may be times when, as you are allowing a PCD to express themselves, you are not sure of the *semantic intent* or specifically what they are attempting to convey. The *semantic intent* is clear when you understand and know what is being said. Often, a PCD will make a statement to me that will sound clear, but I may not always "get it." That is when I "*recreate the conversation.*" I might add that my listening skills have also improved because I *recreate a conversation* any time I am unsure of the semantic intent.

The first way to go about recreating a conversation is to acknowledge what the person said to you, or what you thought they said, especially if you had some difficulty following its intent. In this instance you may have listened to many statements made, and if you are unsure, you might say something like the following: "Okay, Annette. What I get so far is that you just got a new phone, and your son wanted to borrow it. You let him, and now you are upset because you allowed him to do so. Is that right?"

Most PCDs like it when you *recreate a conversation*, especially if you are not 100 percent certain of what they wanted to convey to you. They realize that you want to understand them, rather than giving them half-hearted acknowledgement that you understand what they said when you really didn't. One of the most discourteous things a listener can do when speaking with a PCD is to *acknowledge that you understood what was said when you really did not!*

Another way to recreate a conversation is to request that the PCD give you statements, one at a time. You will do this in a case where the language formulation is skewed, or if the speech intelligibility is severe. The SM attempts to understand what was said, one statement at a time, and put its content back into a simple *Embedded Question* and *Tell Me Phrase* that will be easier to for the PCD to say. The person with the speaking difficulty will then express each statement with clarity since you took the time to put the content into a question and tell me phrase in a manageable bite-sized piece. You would use this second method with those who may have more trouble with language formulation or speech intelligibility, such as those with dysarthria.

Example

SM: Okay, Annette. This is what I get: You just got a new phone?

PCD: Yeah.

SM: YES?

PCD: YES.

PCD: Tell me you got a new phone, using "I."

SM: I GOT A NEW PHONE.

SM: And your son borrowed it?

PCD: YES.

SM: Tell me your son borrowed it, using "my."

PCD: MY SON BORROWED IT.

SM: And you let him.

PCD: YEAH.

SM: Tell me you let him, using "I." Say: I LET HIM.

PCD: I LET HIM.

SM: And now you are mad?

PCD: YEAH, MAD.

SM: So you are mad?

SM: Say: I AM MAD.
PCD: I AM MAD.
SM: Mad at yourself?
PCD: YEAH. MAD AT MYSELF.

Do you see that this is a conversation that soon takes off like it has a "life of its own," which it does! You never get this "live action, in the moment" content for language stimulation from worksheets and repeating prepackaged phrases taken from a computer or speech exercise workbook. This is what a conversation is all about, what human communication is about. We move into *stimulated conversation* as soon as a person is capable of answering questions with regularity. It will happen for you, too, if you have the right mix. The right mix of what? Potential, determination, and playing full out! Stimulated conversation occurs when your PCD gets accustomed to answering *Embedded Questions* and *Tell Me Phrases*. When you have any difficulty understanding or following a communicative interaction with the PCD, recreate the conversation by telling the PCD what you understood. As you repeat in simple phrases or sentences what you understood, watch for the *Yes/No* physiology. When you have the *intent* of it, pause. At this point, you can restimulate the conversation by going through each step again, drawing out correct language usage by asking *Embedded Questions* and using *Tell Me Phrases*.

I will give you one more example. Remember that when PCDs begin to speak again, there will be times when they get confused or forget what they were saying, or they may make paraphasic errors. If while you are listening to them, you find what they are saying hard to follow, I would pursue *The Shadowing Method*.

The Shadowing Method

The Shadowing Method can be used to assure accurate language formulation and comprehension within the conversation. As the PCD starts to regain the ability to formulate language independently, they may tend to speak in a hurry, or rush themselves and speak in more than one sentence. This may create havoc with the listener since it will often disrupt speech intelligibility and the *semantic intent*, the meaning of what the person is attempting to convey. If this should happen to you in your communicative interaction, I suggest that you do the following:

As you listen to each phrase and sentence, stop the forward movement of the conversation and say, *"I want to make sure that I completely understand everything you want to say to me. Therefore, I am going to repeat after you everything you say so that I completely understand what you want to tell me. And if you want, I can help you say what you just said again so that your speech will get even clearer and better!"* Telling them this will really score brownie points with the PCD, since you are conveying two very important messages to them: (1) You want to understand everything they say, and (2) you are going to do everything humanly possible to help them speak with better clarity. When you convey that, you will have a very happy and excited person to work with, and a much deeper relationship or friendship forever. I know this from experience.

Example

SM:	Okay, Annette. I understand that you got a new phone. Tell me again, you got a new phone.
PCD:	I GOT A NEW PHONE.
SM:	And then what?
PCD:	HE TAKE.
SM:	He took it home?
PCD:	HE TOOK IT HOME.
SM:	It's your phone, right?
PCD:	YEAH.
SM:	Whose phone?
PCD:	MINE.
SM:	Tell me: IT'S MY PHONE!
PCD:	IT'S MY PHONE!
SM:	Not his phone, right?
PCD:	YEAH.
SM:	Not his phone?
PCD:	NOT HIS PHONE.
SM:	It's yours.
PCD:	YES.
SM:	Tell me: IT'S MINE!
PCD:	IT'S MINE.
SM:	What's yours?
PCD:	PHONE.
SM:	Tell me: THE PHONE ➔ IS MINE.
PCD:	THE PHONE ➔ IS MINE.
SM:	You need that phone, right?

PCD: YES.

SM: Tell me: I NEED ➜ THE PHONE.

PCD: I NEED ➜ THE PHONE.

SM: Do you want the phone back?

PCD: YES.

SM: Tell him: I WANT ➜ MY PHONE.

PCD: I WANT ➜ MY PHONE!

SM: Will you do that, Annette; when you see him? Tell him: I WANT ➜ MY PHONE.

PCD: YES. I WANT ➜ MY PHONE.

What you are doing here is intentionally recreating each sentence uttered by the PCD from the example in *Recreating a Conversation* shown above, where Annette attempts to say many sentences, the sounds disintegrate and the formulation of words becomes difficult. This keeps the PCD from moving on with forward velocity. When you see speech begin to deteriorate, return the conversation to a single sentence level, so that they have more conscious control over the formulation of words and the articulation of the sounds within those words. Remember that slower speed for those with speaking difficulties often gives them greater control of language formulation and motor speech. You, as the SM, provide the model for the new sounds, words, speed, and manner of speaking, which is totally unlike the way they spoke before. For the child or person who is just learning to speak, the same holds true: you, as the SM, model the sounds, words, speed, and grammar of the talking. This should be done slowly.

You will have opportunities to recreate conversations as your PCDs begin to express themselves. You can either follow the *Recreating a Conversation Method,* allowing them to make a few statements to get the gist of their *semantic intent,* and then walk them through what you were able to glean from their statements, stimulating phrases and sentences in the process; or you can use the *Shadowing Method,* and ask them to tell you what they want to say one sentence at a time. As the SM, you can then clarify what you heard while you improve the structure and clarity of what they said by having them utter the new "updated model."

Conversation Helps Us Determine How We Are Alike and Different

Conversations help us sort out how we are alike and different from the people we meet. We make judgments about whether we would like to have a relationship with a person based on similarities and differences. Imagine what life would be like if we could not communicate verbally with other human beings. We could not share very much, and the result would be isolation. Conversations with others help us to determine if we like that person, and whether we wish to establish a friendship with them.

The other day, my wife and I went to dinner with a new friend of hers. This friend was recently married, and she and my wife wanted the husbands to meet to see if it might be fun doing some social things together. I was told that he was an engineer, and "foreign born." Immediately, I wondered if we would hit it off, since I was already aware of two differences.

We met for dinner, and while I was busy compiling in my mind a list of our similarities and differences, I learned that he had engineered some voice software. Immediately we found something of mutual interest. The conversation quickly focused on software for the speaking voice and some new ways it could be used for therapy. We also talked about voice instrumentation, and new ways it could be used to help people with voice difficulties. All of a sudden, we were *dancing in the conversation*, and at the end of the evening we expressed a desire to get together again socially. I know that with time, we will explore how we can help one another develop new ways to approach therapy. It's all about similarities and differences and finding areas of interest. Conversation affords us that.

What It's like to Stimulate Speech and Language All Day Long

What is it like to stimulate speech all day long? This is an interesting question. Many of us in the field of speech language pathology may know, since we come eye-to-eye with people each day, and are paid to do it. That gives the speech-language pathologist some idea of what it is like. In a way, it reminds me of a particular situation with my mother when I was a young child, whenever a grammatical error was made. She would ceaselessly correct me by saying what the proper grammatical form was. For instance, I always had a problem with the use of objective pronouns, when we refer to ourselves at the end of a sentence in the predicate. I used to say: "Linda is going with me and Paul." My mother would then say, "You mean, 'Linda is going with Paul and me?'" And of course I would then say, "Yes, Linda is going with me and Paul." She would correct me again and say, "Yes, Linda is going with Paul and me," until finally I got it right. She would do that any time she heard an error; and, before long, I spoke with exceptional grammar.

I used to say, "Me and her are going." My mother would quickly ask the question and say, "You mean, 'She and I are going?'" Then I would correctly say: "Yes, Mom, 'she and I are going,'" followed by rolling my eyes up at the ceiling and saying, "Okay, Mom!" In a way, I really didn't like her correcting me, but I knew I had to say it right. This is what it will be like for you, should you decide to truly commit to this way of thinking, doing, and stimulating speech and language.

Believe me, it is a commitment to really take a stand and constantly stimulate speech and language all day long, but that is what it will take if you are truly going to help the PCD. For the caregiver, it will be a totally different experience to be stimulating correct speech and language "all day long," especially when, prior to this training, you have done it in a way that may or may not have been readily accepted by the PCD. Most caregivers and spouses have no clue about how to stimulate speech and language with a person who once had the ability to speak, or with an individual who never learned to speak. Quite often, it is very frustrating to everyone involved, since few really know what to do to help the PCD speak correctly. You will be one of the select few who develops the ability to stimulate talking with those who cannot.

What an enrolling conversation about
The Teaching of Talking might look and sound like

When I pursued Landmark Education a few years ago, I learned about "Enrolling Conversations." I adapted this concept to the idea of "getting permission" from the PCD to stimulate their speech all day long. It is a conversation in which you as a speech-language pathologist or caregiver, have a discussion with the PCD to determine whether he or she is willing to make a personal commitment to better speech and language, or "talking." You enter the world of the person with the speaking difficulty, and determine whether they are "up" for doing whatever it takes for speech improvement to occur.

This type of conversation requires personal power and persuasion on the part of the SM, in addition to at least two other crucial communicative abilities: the power of rapport and courtesy in conversation. An enrolling conversation is one in which you speak from your heart in a way that is truly intended. This level of sincerity is essential when you are having a conversation with the person who has the speaking difficulty in order to obtain their permission to engage them in the expression and expansion of their speech and language –a process that YOU will be helping them to accomplish.

Remember that conventional speech and language therapy will hardly be enough stimulation for the majority of people with moderate to profound communication difficulty. Their progress in speech and language therapy will be much faster if there is a committed caregiver who is willing to learn the methods of *The Teaching of Talking*, a considerable task in itself, and who is also willing to *take a stand* to use it throughout the day to model correct speech and language, and to require a spoken response. In that way, both of you will know there is improvement each and every time words are spoken, and you will both note improvement on an hourly, daily, weekly, monthly, and yearly basis.

Therefore, the enrolling conversation is held between the caregiver or SM and the PCD to assure that there is agreement and commitment to this process. The chances are favorable for the desired results when there is *agreement and mutual commitment for improved speech*. Both of these are essential.

The person with the speaking difficulty *must want speech and language improvement*, and that is another *foundation stone of the work* — a true desire by the PCD and the SM for improved communication.

The other day, I was working with a man and his wife in speech and language therapy. She was disappointed that her husband often did not want to respond when she asked him questions throughout the day pertaining to things that he might want to eat or do. She stated that it was frustrating for her, since he did not always seem to be "cooperating." He too rolled his eyes toward the ceiling, just like I used to do when my mother "corrected" me. I knew that I had similar feelings in response to my mother when she was correcting or "stimulating" my grammar as a boy. I therefore understood his position.

To continue with my story, I was doing speech and language stimulation with a gentleman and his wife, and she informed me that her husband had not been very cooperative. I knew that she was relatively competent in this method, as they had been coming to therapy for about eight weeks. You just can't expect much improvement if the PCD and SM are not in conversation, stimulating expressive speech and language. At this point in my career, I do not want to spend a lot of time with people who are not committed to doing what it takes to get the job done! Therefore, the three of us had a conversation that went something like this:

SM: Now John, I need to ask you a question. Do you like therapy?

PCD: Yes.

SM: Tell me: I LIKE THERAPY.

PCD: I LIKE THERAPY.

SM: Do you want to talk?

PCD: Yes.

SM: Tell me: I WANT TO TALK.

PCD: I WANT TO TALK.

SM: Now, John, I hate to waste your time and mine, and what I hear you saying is that you like therapy.

SM: Tell me: I LIKE THERAPY.

PCD: I LIKE THERAPY.

SM: You want to talk?

SM: Yes.

PCD: Tell me: I WANT TO TALK.

PCD: WANT TO TALK.

SM: WHO WANTS TO TALK?

PCD: I WANT TO TALK.

SM: So you like therapy?

PCD: I LIKE THERAPY.

SM: AND YOU WANT TO TALK?

PCD: I WANT TO TALK.

SM: So you like therapy?

PCD: I LIKE THERAPY.

SM: And you want to talk?

PCD: I WANT TO TALK.

SM: John, You must talk all the time. Do you get that?

PCD: I GET THAT.

SM: So you want to talk?

PCD: YES.

SM: Tell me you want to talk.

PCD: I WANT TALK.

SM: Tell me you want ➜ to talk.

PCD: I WANT ➜ TO TALK.

SM: All the time?

PCD: Yes.

SM: Tell me: ALL THE TIME.

PCD: ALL THE TIME.

SM: What was that?

PCD: ALL THE TIME.

SM: And you want to talk all the time?

PCD: YES.

SM: Tell me you want to talk all the time.

PCD: I WANT TO TALK ALL THE TIME.

SM: Tell me again?

PCD: I WANT TO TALK →ALL THE TIME.

The conversation now starts to become more generative and especially geared to John's level of communicative difficulty. It is short and sweet, and constantly stimulating the formation and expression of language and confirming we each understand the intent of the other. At this point in John's therapy, the *Tell Me Phrase* does not always have to be fully expressed by the SM. After a while, the PCD picks up the language from the initial question and the *Tell Me Phrase* can be phased out of the conversation. However, when needed, it can be readily reinserted. When it comes to the expression of language, we all have days that are better than others. On some days, you will need to use the *Tell Me Phrase*, and on other days it won't be necessary.

The following conversation was meant for John's wife, but spoken to John. This was a conversation that she thought was directed to John. Now, this conversation was really on the rather difficult side for John, since it was spoken at a rate and complexity appropriate for John's wife. She thought I was speaking to him, but in reality I was speaking to her. The conversation is a metaphor, and it is really about the caregiver's commitment to the person they are with. It is filled with indirect suggestions for his wife and all about commitment and regularity. I know it takes two people to have a conversation, and both individuals must take equal responsibility to make it happen, just like doing and succeeding in therapy. Whether John got this was not the intention; the intention was that his wife *heard*, and understood me, and applied what she heard.

Now if you truly wish to get better, John, will you agree to answer your wife's questions, even if you don't want to? We both know there are lots of things in life that we don't want to do, but we know we must do them if we are going to succeed. I know you know that. I didn't really want to get out of bed this morning, but I knew that I had to, or I wouldn't be here to help you, and I would not get paid. And the same thing goes for you when you really don't feel like talking or answering her questions or asking for things at home. You know that if you don't speak throughout the day, your speech won't improve, and you know that coming to speech therapy two to three times a week is just not going to cut the mustard. It's just not going to do what you think it will do for you. Your real improvement will come when you talk at home when questions are asked of you and you answer them – even if you don't want to!

Now, John, I'd like to tell you a story about my wife, Malka. She has been in this country for a little bit over a year, and when she came here she could not speak a lick of English. Like you with your speaking right now, I told Malka that I would help her speak and that I would be stimulating her speech all day long if she wished, and Malka said that was fine. Now, I can't believe it, John. I am constantly restimulating Malka's speech and constantly expanding what she says and correcting her grammar and vocabulary choices and pronunciation all day long, and you know something, John? She never minds me doing that. I keep waiting for the time when Malka will tell me to "go jump in the lake," but she always responds with correct speech and grammar to my questions or Tell Me Phrases. I show her the right way to say something and then stimulate it throughout the day, and now she is speaking better and better. She is the only person I know who takes my suggestions just about every time I give them! You too will improve your speaking, John, if you can just agree to allow Joan to ask you the questions and you say the phrases and sentences.

I realize, John, that Malka really wants to speak the language, and will do just about anything to make that happen. Do you REALLY want to improve your ability to speak, and will you do whatever you can to answer our questions with phrases and sentences? I know you will improve your speaking because you already have in the short period of time we have been working. You know that, right?

And there's the rub. If you can get the PCD to *buy in,* you can get the PCD and SM back into a conversation that can continue all day long, one that will be a healthy process, so long as both people are committed to the idea. I know what it is like to stimulate patients all day long and then go home and do it all evening and weekend long. And, dear reader, there will be times when you may be tired, or fed up, or question whether the person you are with will truly improve. The principles of *persistence* and *perseverance* are as vital for the caregiver as they are for the PCD. Persist, and continue to do what you know will bring improvement in speaking for the person you are stimulating.

Even when I feel like giving myself or Malka a rest from speech and language stimulation, I persevere, because in truth, it doesn't take a lot more effort to stimulate speech than not. Just go ahead and do it, and you will both reap the rewards. Others will see speaking improvement because you hung in there, just like Helen Keller, who had an intense desire to express spoken language and pursued it for most of her life. An old friend of mine by the name of Dr. Gregory Cheatwood used to say, *You can't row a person across the river without getting over to the other side yourself.*

Go for it with gusto, and realize you will get the results if you, the SM, and the PCD are in agreement about pursuing therapy. If there is no agreement, only conflict or resistance, the results will not be satisfactory.

> "I once learned that if you can express what your intention is and why, and if you are honest and speak from the heart, then others, who are desirous of change will, chances are, understand your sincerity and acquiesce."
>
> —Ittleman

What Does It Take to Succeed and How Long Does it Take?

Once you understand how to stimulate a response by using an *Embedded Question, Alternate Choice, a Tell Me Phrase,* a *What It is©* Statement, or a *"I'll Tell You about Me, and You Tell Me about You"* procedure, you will be well under way to learning how to do remarkable speech and language stimulation in conversation, without all the copied handouts. You will be ready to have a conversation without spending time in a panic looking for an exercise out of one of the aphasia handbooks, or spending time at the copier, copying meaningless drivel that no one really cares about, since it has little or no meaning to the person with whom you are speaking.

I developed and authored a program for people with aphasia who had lost their ability to speak. It was designed with one question in mind: "What kind of treatment would you give people with severe to profound Broca's-like aphasia *if there were no constraints?*" I wanted to create something unconventional. I knew what the results were like when conventional therapy was given two to three times a week in a small therapy cubicle with pencil or pen and ink drawings. I hammered out what the picture of speech and language stimulation would look like if there were "no constraints."

I believe that frequency of speech and language therapy is important. "When discussing therapy for adult apraxics or children with developmental apraxia, Campbell, Rosenbek and others agree that patients and clinicians should have daily sessions."[-18]

After providing intensive daily therapy five times a week, eight hours per day, to four adult patients with severe to profound expressive aphasia and apraxias with two CNAs and family volunteers, I realized that the process of language stimulation was an ongoing process that should not even be thought about in terms of frequency or length of treatment. After three years of providing daily speech therapy for eight hours a day, I came to the conclusion that for profound Broca's-like aphasia and other profound communication problems that are neurologically based, it was best to *concentrate on the speech and language stimulation.* The responsibility for getting better, or having a return of functional speech, would be better left to *G-d*[19], chance, and the individuals' proclivity for making what is desired happen! I cannot state it more simply. I have colleagues who may argue about specific numbers of thirty or sixty minute sessions with a CCC Speech-Language Pathologist, or about site of lesion and other neurological lingo; but, to me, it's a crap-shoot. Many factors may never even be measureable, such as the role of the clinician and his or her ability to inspire and motivate the patients, or the intensity of the therapy, the personal or intellectual disposition of each participant and of the therapist, and the type of therapy provided.

Qualities of the Speech Model

So what does it take to succeed? First, I believe it is, in part, the charisma and confidence of the person who stimulates the speech and language, and whether they are personally likeable or focused enough to keep the person with the speaking difficulty in the conversation. This particular quality involves a personal

---

18 Thomas F. Campbell., "Functional Treatment Outcomes in Young Children with Motor Speech Disorders," In Clinical Management of Motor Speech Disorders in Children, edited by Anthony J. Caruso and Edythe A. Strand, 394 (New York: Thieme Medical Publishers Inc., 1999).

19 This word is not misspelled; it is spelled this way out of respect for the author's religious traditions.

intensity and an ability to engage the individual. The rest of the qualities have been alluded to earlier in this text, and would be worthy of your review.

Qualities of the Person with the Communication Difficulty

The qualities of the person with the speaking difficulty must include a true desire to improve. The PCD must have a junkyard dog mentality to dig into the language stimulation process and never give up, even if it takes a lifetime. The reason why I believe this therapy works is because there are no barriers regarding what *should* be said, *where* it should be done, *what is or is not* said, or the *frequency* or *intensity* of what is said (I could tell you some stories of words and phrases PCDs have wanted me to stimulate!) I have no intention of dictating a protocol to anyone, especially since most people do what they darned well want to do anyway. My message here is for you to become aware of the richness of spoken language every day, no matter where you are. Every opportunity to speak and communicate is the realm where we must encourage and provide speech and language stimulation for the person who is halted in the ability to talk, and to stimulate them to speak in the easiest and most enjoyable manner, not with practice sheets that are designed for children, or with people who have diametrically opposed interests or values. It is *our responsibility to identify the interests and values of each person* with whom we are working, and then use that information within speaking opportunities to stimulate speech, in a manner that will easily yield to the expression of speaking.

If you were to ask me how long it takes to help the individual with a severe to profound speaking difficulty, or how often a PCD may need therapy, especially if it was related to stroke, I would say it generally takes years of speech and language stimulation in the context of daily living, at home or wherever the person is, and having someone available to constantly challenge them to speak. Helen Keller, who was deaf and blind, was a prime example. She had Ann Sullivan stimulate her with finger spelling into her palm, learning Braille and spoken language for hours and hours each day, year after year. Ann Sullivan was Helen's governess and teacher for twenty years, and then her companion for another twenty years.

Anne Sullivan arrived at Keller's house in March 1887, and immediately began to teach Helen to communicate by spelling words into her hand, beginning with "d-o-l-l" for the doll that she had brought Keller as a present. Keller was frustrated, at first, because she did not understand that every object had a word uniquely identifying

it. In fact, when Sullivan was trying to teach Keller the word for "doll,"
Keller became so frustrated she broke the doll. Keller's big breakthrough
in communication came the next month, when she realized that the
motions her teacher was making on the palm of her hand, while
running cool water over her other hand, symbolized the idea of
"water"! She then nearly exhausted Sullivan demanding the names of
all the other familiar objects in her world.[20]

Keller said the moment "awakened (her) soul" to the potential
for her life. She later became an internationally celebrated writer and
advocate for those with disabilities. She died in 1968.[21]

It is a real treat now for me to read the insightful writings of Helen Keller, who was curious, highly educated, and a worldwide traveler. She was also very interested in politics and advocacy for public policies.

It is too bad that there are many people today, whose lives have been interrupted by a traumatic event that may be temporarily robbing them of the ability to comprehend or to speak, who resort to staying at home, doing nothing but eating, sleeping, and watching TV. I encourage you to engage the person who has a speaking difficulty, and do not allow them to retreat into the *closet of life*. Encourage speaking at every opportunity for both the person who has not developed speech automatically and for those who may have temporarily lost the ability due to a traumatic episode. You can do it! Come with me and I will show you.

---

20   Wikipedia, The Free Encyclopedia, accessed May 2011, http://en.wikipedia.org/Helen%20Keller.
21   "Helen Keller Statue Unveiled in Capitol, First Statue Honoring Disabled Person in U.S. Capitol Replaces Statue of Confederate Veteran." The Associated Press, Washington D.C., September 7, 2009.

The Tools of the Trade: What Every Speech-Language Pathologist and Speech Model Should Have at Their Disposal

As previously mentioned, I had a professor at the University of Miami in Coral Gables, Florida (1968-1971), who repeatedly reminded us that *an exceptional clinician should be able to do a communication assessment and therapy with tools as simple as a pen and a legal pad.* That was forty years ago! At that time, we used audio recorders; and standardized tests were just emerging, many of them without "norms." During the early 1970s, more and more tests were developed with normative data. Some of the researchers at that time, such as Lois Bloom, were reporting data in language development from painstaking documentation of their children's speech and language development.

For many years, it was my personal ambition to satisfy the challenge of one of my mentors, Dr. Jack Bensen, head of the speech therapy clinic in the '60s and '70s at the University of Miami, who emphasized the necessity of normative data for research and documentation and to ensure that we as a profession demonstrate competence within our education and health care institutions. I concur with his challenge even today.

But what about getting an accurate measurement of the progress of an individual's development of speech and language competency based on what he or she is able to say in a normal conversation? Another one of my mentors,

Dr. Thomas Shriner, who was an editor for JSHR (the Journal of Speech and Hearing Research), was instrumental in instilling in us the discipline to look at speech and language competence by measuring the speech output in terms of articulation, language, grammar, syntax, and morphology from a formal language sample. Is the person's standard score on a testing instrument or verbal age equivalent significant in the approach to therapy? Probably not. Is it one of the ways to document the efficacy of therapy to government, insurance, health and educational institutions? The author pleads the fifth.[22]

The Personal Laptop or Computer

Current technology has been very instrumental in providing tools for the speech-language pathologist or caregiver when stimulating language. Although the legal pad can still be helpful in a pinch, the computer or iPad devices now available, being light and portable, have many wonderful uses.

Documentation and Therapy

The personal computer is instrumental in the documentation of speech and language assessment. The speech and language output can be recorded on a digital or video recorder and then, with periodic assessments at weekly or monthly intervals, one can ascertain any change in communicative function. In the assessment forms at many hospitals today, percentage scores are reported for immediate, short-term memory, auditory recognition, discrimination, cognitive scores, and other assessments. Percentages and normative data continue to be essential for evaluation and documentation.

The tool that is most *evidence-based* is a videotape recorder, which can show the true evidence of improvement and a transcribed language sample on a word processing program, along with a phonetic record and intelligibility scores to track improvement in language competence, articulation, motor speech, and dysarthria. Reporting voice improvement is an excellent form of documentation, especially to compare the habitual voice at start of care while reading a reading passage and in conversation with a reporting of the parameters of the speaking voice, i.e., *decibels, Hz, vocal quality, resonance, and tone focus.*

---

22 The legal phrase "to plead the fifth" has also entered common vernacular. In a casual setting, you may hear people say they plead the fifth when asked something because their answer might be incriminating or simply something they don't want to divulge. http://www.wisegeek.com/what-does-it-mean-to-plead-the-fifth.htm.

In recent years, SLPs have been called on to justify their treatment decisions with sound scientific evidence and have been seeking resources to effectively engage in evidence-based practice (EBP). Originating from a definition by Sackett and colleagues,[23] EBP refers to "the integration of best research evidence with clinical expertise and client values." EBP informs clinicians who seek the best treatment course based on a balance between research-based evidence, clinical expertise and experience, and the client's wishes. Providers evaluate the scientific literature as it pertains to the choice of a specific diagnostic protocol or treatment approach.[24]

I like simplicity. The computer is useful to print a clear and readable document that attests to the speech and language competence of the individual.

It is the opinion of this author that the measurement of evidence-based practice (EBP) is the answer to the following questions:

- *Is the PCD speaking better (as evidenced by MLU, language sample; complexity of language, grammatical intricacy; or accuracy of articulation)?*
- *Is he or she more readily understood?*
- *Is the intelligibility of speaking better?*

Do you remember the early language samples of Ray on page 17? This is the language sample taken over a year later. To me, this shows true progress of speech and language competence, rather than looking at statistical scores from standardized tests.

I been up at 2 am.
I drank coffee.
I had 3 and a half cups and I ate breakfast.
I had a eggs toast.
And then I fed Jim-Bo.
I got up Sally.
Terrible.
I got dressed.

---

23   David Sackett, "What is Evidence-Based Practice (EBP)," UNC Health Sciences Library, 1996, accessed October 2011, http://www.hsl.unc.edu/services/tutorials/ebm/whatis.htm.

24   Tobi Frymark MA, and Carol Smith Hammond, Ph.D. "Guest Editorial: Evidence-Based Practice and Speech-Language Pathology," accessed October 2011, Journal of Rehabilitation Research & Development. Vol. 46. no. 2. (2009), http://www.rehab.research.va.gov/jour/09/46/2/index.html.

Then let Jim-Bo out, and then I headed for Houston.
We left the house at 6:30 am.
I fixed her a grilled cheese sandwich.
She drank water.
I am. I barely got here in time to use the bathroom.
Andrew he picks me up around 5:20.
6:30.
We are late.
I went to bed at 8:00 pm.
Tell her that David Letterman can wait.
David Letterman comes on at 10:30 pm.
I got up to go to the bathroom and she was not in bed yet.
And it was 11 o'clock.
That TV she was watching was in the den.
When I go to bed, I go to bed. No TV!
David Letterman is over at 11:30.
I don't know; I be sleeping.
Sally made me mad yesterday.
I needed validation whether supper was good.
I cooked all the meals.
And nothing......
She didn't say thank you and I cooked a roast with new potatoes.
I shouldn't have to?
That fine but I don't want my ass to be chewed out.
That would be too easy.
For me.
I went to bed.
But I cooked her Parker House rolls.
You know what a Parker House roll?
In aluminum pan; bake them.
She ate 4 of them.
I had 2.
I cooked a half a pan.
She is on a diet.
It was good.

The dishes were stacked in the sink.
I have to load the dishwasher.
I use an iron pot.
Cast iron

Most people have iPads, laptops, and personal computers in this day and age. The computer is an excellent device to use as an adjunct tool in the stimulation of speech and language. Stimulation of speech requires cues, or ways to get the person to utter sounds or words. In many cases, we as SMs will utter a sound or word, and the PCD will repeat or imitate it. With time and practice the SM learns the words, phrases, and length of sentence the PCD can say without difficulty.

Sometimes, in addition to *saying* the stimulus words for the PCD, it is helpful to type them in a large font on a computer screen that is strategically placed in front of the PCD. Remember that you want to be sitting across from the PCD to stimulate him or her at approximately three to five feet, very much like looking into a mirror and seeing yourself. In this way, the PCD can readily hear you, read your lips, and simultaneously or separately see the extra-large font on the computer screen displaying what you want them to say. You can simultaneously print the sound, word, phrase, or sentence that you wish the PCD to say as you are having him say it. You can also use the printed word to help the person who may have an apraxia of speech, especially emphasizing phonemes or sounds they may be having difficulty with. Those persons with speaking difficulties (PSDs.) may also have difficulty saying multi-syllable words, and specific speech sounds. The personal computer could be used in these instances to print out the syllables of words and break down the word into simple units of speech, which can then be approached in bite sized pieces. For example:

(street: sssssss ➜ tah ➜reet), or (barbecue: bar ➜ bah ➜ ka ➜ you)

The other nice thing about a computer such as a laptop or an iPad is that a PCD can keep lists of words that you have covered in a Word Document. The words can be individually transliterated for the PCD to say, and can also be placed in alphabetical order for quick reference.

Articulation and Pronunciation List

afford	ah-----for-----d	Lexus	Leck------sus
answered	an-- ---sir---t	mechanic	ma—ka—nik
black	ba---lack	napkins	nap---kins
blades	ba---lades	onions	un---yen
bleeder	ba----leeder	ordered	or---der---t
blue	ba---lou	part	parrrrrrrrrr---t
bread	ba---red	please	pa---leeeeeez
brought	ba---raw---t	plenty	pa---lenty
brown	ba---rown	queen	ka---ween
catsup	catch---up	replace	re- pa---lace
Charlie	char---lee	Ro-tel	row---tell
Christmas	kah---riss---mass	scare	Sa-----care
clock	ka---lock	second	Se------kint
crumb	ka---rums	security	sah---cure---ah---tee
Dennis	den-----nissss	sleep	s-----leeeeeeep
drink	da---rink	sleepy	s------leeeee---pee
drive	da---rive	slept	s-----lep----t
freeze	fa---reez	slippers	s---lip—pers
fried	fa---rye-d	slow	sa---low
fries	fa rye----s	smoked	sa---mowk---t
frozen	fa---row---zen	smothered	ssss---mother—t
garage	ga rah----sh	social	sew---shell
gravy	ga---ravy	spell	sssss----pell
gripe	ga---ripe	stay	sssss-----tay
ground	ga---round	street	S-----ta---reet
groves	ga-----rowv----s	strength	ssss---ta---ren—th
handkerchief	hang—ker-chiff	stuff	ssss----tuff
Hebrew	he---ba---rew	Therapist	ther---ahhhhh---piss--t
husband	huz---band	Track	ta---rack
job	sneeze J---ob		

Start of Care	3-Month Language Sample	6-Month Language Sample	9-Month Language Sample	15-Month Language Sample	18-Month Language Sample
I tut rat and wee eetid. (I cut grass and weed eated.)	I ----- senk 4 uh uh coffee. (I drink 4 cups of coffee.)	She says I have to brin her out to eash lunch (She says I have to bring her out to eat lunch)	I don't know ih I tell you any ting.	I got up at 3:30	Sally is in Austin
A tee sop (at the shop)	No.	Papa seetas… in hews ton…on… innertate… sten (Pappasitos in Houston on Interstate 10)	No lan wont come any way.	I didn't drink coffee	She is be home tonight
She hant haw afor me. (She can't afford me.)	I work (I worked)	I maze ayds tot. I mase ayd toas. (I made egg toast)	No lan would not come any way.	Miss Mary she gave me @ $200.00 for my birthday	She is going to be home tonight
No.	I wort at sepis taytin (I worked at a service station)	I have thee eds (I had 3 eggs)	Cawt…he don't like my cut tin (Cause he don't like my cooking)	Save it.	Shopping

I don't want to tut tas. (I don't want to cut grass.)	Huf (Gulf)	Cuz she kin int deh uh (Because she couldn't get up)	I in vite him o ber for beer ssssss pa raw gin off (I invited him over for beef stroginoff)	Miss Mary	Herself
I soo. (I do.)	I humph hass (I pumped gas)	I got hup at thee A M (I got up at 3 AM)	I in vite him ohder faw beef sssssssss tah raw in off and he didin come (I invited him over for beef stroganoff and he didn't come)	Sally wrote e mails	Yeah
She mase me sim and all. (She makes me??)	I wat tisteen (I was sixteen)	She kinint het up at 5 am (She couldn't get up at 5 am)	He had aw dehdee bot tih kin (he had already bought chicken)	You wrote 2 e mails	Yeah

Is on huh (??)	Tah der (dollar)		Tarita tah…set… at…No… lan would buy chi len (Theresa said that No lan would buy chicken)	I wrote the first one	Sally, she brought her sister
	I was matin a dah der (I was makin a dollar)		I woud know (I wouldn't know)	I can't believe!	She rode with her
	I was wortin to mate a buck (??)		No lan bought fries cah fiss (Ar ture bought fried cat fish)	I went to Dairy Queen and I saw 3 buddies of mine	Sally's sister Julia
	I wuh nun no (I wouldn't know)		I lite fied cah fiss (I like fried cat fish)	And they didn't understand what I said	They do nothing but shop
				They were 3 buddy of mine from total	Cindy, talked to Javier about my blower

				I get in ta rouble (trouble) for	Cindy, talked to Javier about my blower
				TAW—KING (talking)	Javier said he was coming in three weeks
				I fik--- sssssss dinner on Sunday	Javier is going to fix my blower
				Beef sssss-ta – aw ---- kin off	I bought another one
				Ba ra ka lee (broccoli)	My new blower cost one hundred and fifty dollars
				And Parker- House rolls	Give it to the George
				We are going to have for dinner tonight	Yeah
				I ssssaid guess what we are having tonight	George has a house in Nederland

					Leftovers .... Beef	George he have a house in Nederland
					I thank Sally for bringing me	I don't know
					I have no money	I am mighty fine
					$500.00 you spend	I bought a battery for my car
					I invited them to dinner	I bought at Sears, it was a die hard
					George and Ka ris see	My battery cost one hundred dollars
						While the mouse is away, I will play
						While the mouse is away, I will play
						Saturday
						Last Saturday

If you are working on an expressive language exercise, you can transcribe the exercise you are doing at the same time as you are stimulating speech. Make sure the PCD is able to pick up cues from written words, as some may have an alexia, or difficulty with the recognition of printed single words, phrases or sentences.

Example

I want → to go to_____.

> the doctor
> therapy
> the post office
> mail box

As the SM reviews this grammatical structure, the PCD sees, hears, and feels the spoken sentence through the different senses, so that it gets through to the brain more readily. When this occurs, learning the grammatical structure is faster, because you are using the input modalities of sight, hearing, and motor programming.

A Video and Voice Recording Device for Documentation and Therapy

Improvements in technology are constant. Video and voice recording devices can now fit in one's shirt pocket, and the images and audio quality are excellent. The smart phones today have built in cameras, HD video recording devices and audio sound bites that can be recorded in a session and e-mailed to the client's home when the session is concluded.

I now record initial assessments, and periodically record the patients' speech at regular intervals. It is amazing to play back recordings and compare language samples of individuals who have been receiving speech and language stimulation for many months. With these devices in hand, anyone can plainly see changes in speech and language performance. The results will speak for themselves and will add additional credence to sole numbers, standard scores, and percentages. Documenting improvement with these devices should be used with increasing regularity by all those in the field of speech language pathology. If one were to compare videotapes of the same patient over time, one could see a number of remarkable changes that would give more backbone to numerical scores reported.

1. A comparison of the ability to speak at the end versus the start of care (videotape and language sample)
2. Speech rate comparisons

3. Vocal intensity, quality, resonance, tone focus and optimal pitch of the speaking voice
4. Mean Length Utterance (MLU) –that is, the average number of words uttered per verbal response taken from at least 50 utterances
5. Frequency of anomia and verbal paraphasic errors
   a. percentage of self-recovery without cues
   b. ability to self-edit when errors naturally occur in spoken language
   c. average latency of time to recover the act of speaking when the patient is groping for a word, concept, phrase or sentence (can be measured with or without cues given by the SM.)
6. Expanse of expressive vocabulary and complexity of syntax and grammar

Digital Photography and Immediate Printout Photographs

The literature has clearly demonstrated that stimulus material pertinent to the individual (their house, car, children, family, interests, daily routine, places they visit each day, week, month, or year) are all excellent for stimulating language when an individual is unable to do so in that context and at that moment. PCDs and their caregivers and families can have a great deal of fun photographing a person's daily routine, from the time they get up and throughout the day until it is bedtime. These photographs are usually fun to review, especially at the office of the speech-language pathologist, since he or she is typically unavailable to come to the PCD's house to track what they are doing and saying throughout the day. Photographs should be taken and classified according to categories, such as:

1. Clothing
2. Daily routine
3. Places you go
4. Food that you like
5. Clothing you like to wear
6. People you love
7. How you feel
8. Things that you want and need
9. Money
10. Numbers
11. Hobbies and objects associated with them

12. Favorite places in the house
13. Favorite furniture
14. Tasks that need to be done with regularity at the house
15. Friends
16. Things to do that are fun
17. Restaurants to go to
18. Places to go in town
19. Doctors' offices, staff members and the doctor him/herself
20. Things that must be bought on a regular basis
21. List of objects within each room of the house

Photographs may or may not be as useful to the PCD at home, since they can be speaking there in the context of the situation. Furthermore, during daily outings and activities, these concepts can be stimulated by words, phrases, and sentences in each context. Photographs do help the speech-language pathologist follow what specific language utterances are being stimulated at home, and they give all concerned the opportunity to demonstrate competence in stimulating speech and language, especially in the office. This will help the speech pathologist further understand where additional work is necessary.

One of my favorite patients who comes for therapy is married to a "scrapbooker." She does some beautiful work, and has constructed one of the most wonderful therapy devices that I have ever seen. Per request, she placed a single 4x6 photograph on each page of the scrapbook. Beneath the photograph are three to five simple sentences about the picture. Since this PCD can read single words, phrases and sentences aloud, he can tell us all about the pictures without any *Embedded Questions, Tell Me Phrases, Alternate Choice* or *What It Is*© techniques. He is now able to state many of the phrases spontaneously, without looking at the written words, due to home practice. Researchers in the field of speech language pathology, such as Audrey Holland, PhD., and others, have reported similar findings with their work on script training with aphasia[25], which is similar to memorizing lines or scripts for a play.

The daily review of stimulus materials, such as a scrapbook or computer with written cues, leads the PCD to actually see, hear and feel the language prior to

---

25 " Gina L. Youmans, Audrey L. Holland, and Maria L. Munoz, "Script Training and Automaticity in Two Individuals with Aphasia." accessed 2011, Clinical Aphasiology. http://clinicalaphasiology. org/2004_pdf/Youmans.pdf, 1-5.

speaking in that context. In time the person with the speaking difficulty should begin talking spontaneously.

REVIEW

Computers, video and digital cameras can be instrumental in the measurement and documentation of all aspects of the speech act. They can also be used as clinical tools to facilitate speaking and memory while speech and language stimulation is taking place.

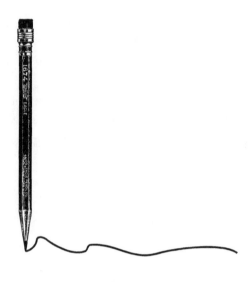

The Concept of
Massed Practice

There is not much more that really needs to be said here. We know that the more one practices anything –if the practicing is done in the correct manner – the greater the likelihood that the behavior will develop. Traditional speech therapy is given two to three times a week and may take place in a group or in individualized treatment for thirty, forty-five, or fifty minute sessions (*distributed practice*). *Massed practice*[26] makes it possible to produce speaking behaviors frequently over a single, prolonged period of time. Traditional speech therapy takes place during a fraction of the individual's waking hours in a clinic, office, or Home Health setting, a few times per week. That is why *The Teaching of Talking* was developed. The frequency and length of duration of most

26 Constraint-Induced Therapy of Chronic Aphasia After Stroke; Taken from *Stroke*. 2001; 32: 1621-1626; @2001 American Heart Association, Inc. Original Contribution Friedemann Pulvermüller, PhD; Bettina Neininger, MA; Thomas Elbert, PhD; Bettina Mohr, PhD; Brigitte Rockstroh, PhD; Peter Koebbel, MA; Edward Taub, PhD. From the MRC Cognition and Brain Sciences Unit (F.P.), Cambridge, UK; Department of Psychology (F.P., B.G., T.E. B.M., B.R.), University of Konstanz, Konstanz; Lurija Institute of Rehabilitation Research (F.P., B.G.); Neurological Hospital Schmieder (P.K.), Allensbach, Germany; and the Department of Psychology (E.T.), University of Alabama at Birmingham, Birmingham, Ala. Correspondence and reprint requests to Friedemann Pulvermüller, Cognition and Brain Sciences Unit, Medical Research Council, 15 Chaucer Rd, Cambridge CB2 2EF, UK.

traditional speech therapy sessions are not enough for the majority of individuals with severe or profound difficulties, and therefore, they do not get the results desired. By training the SM well, *massed practice* is possible at home and during many activities of daily living, every day. Under these circumstances, the PCD should have speech improvement at a faster pace, since he or she is engaged in speaking correctly outside of the clinic or office in activities that are personally interesting and meaningful throughout the day. *Massed practice* is intensive work during a period of time on an idea, concept, word, phrase, or sentence. Distributed practice is similar. However, time elapses between trained speech and language stimulation, usually days. Both massed and distributed practice have been shown to get good results with speech therapy. *The Teaching of Talking* incorporates both concepts, since it facilitates speech when given throughout the day, seven days a week. This is far superior to traditional speech therapy that is done for less than an hour, one to three visits per week. Our method is designed for people who have mild to profound speaking difficulties, which I believe requires intensive stimulation.

Your Approach to Mild Expressive Aphasia

I really did not want to write this chapter; but, alas, I must. You might want to know why.

There are millions of people throughout the United States and the world who have suffered from a stroke or head injury and experienced a disruption in speaking. To them, it is a major challenge. Many engage in conversation only to find they get lost and forget what they said. They may be at a loss for words, or even forget what the other person has said to them. To the speech-language pathologist, this may seem a minor problem to address as compared to their PCDs who are not capable of speaking at all. We, as speech-language pathologists, sometimes do not realize that a minor speaking problem to some people may be as personally devastating as a complete loss of the ability to speak is to someone else.

So then, the question is: "What do I do with one who has a mild disruption of speech, as a professional, spouse, family member, or caregiver? There is often an intermittent anomia, or loss for words, or inability to recall a specifically desired word or thought. This problem may also cause the PCD to get lost in a thought or desired message. This amnesia for a thought happens to us all from time to time. It may occur when we are explaining something and may get interrupted by another thought, or when someone else interrupts us in the middle of thinking or speaking. Anytime you hear someone say, "Now where was I?" the phenomenon of an amnesic episode has just occurred. If lucky, the speaker or listener will recall where they were in the conversation so that it can be continued and concluded.

Therefore, I have included this chapter in *Teaching of Talking* because there are people with mild speaking difficulties who may perceive it as a MAJOR one! Just remember, dear reader, that everything is relative to the individual with the speaking difficulty. Some may look at it as a minor inconvenience, and another as a major life catastrophe.

There are a number of observations you will make about people with expressive aphasia, especially those of the "mild" type. They may include:

1. Intermittent loss for words within the conversation
2. The listener forgets what was said to them just previous, at the end of the conversation or later, after the conversation is completed. The speaker can also forget what they have just said, or later forget the comment made after the conversation.
3. Difficulty communicating with more than one person at a time
4. Difficulty expressing oneself
5. Struggling with thoughts or words
6. Expressing different words than those intended

Having worked with individuals with expressive aphasia for many years, I have some further observations. Many are summed up with an individual I am treating at the present time. I will call him "Gus."

Gus is an individual who owned his own business for many years, and was happily married. After his stroke, he would frequently get confused during conversations and get *stuck* on a thought or word, and would be seemingly unable to complete it. As time progressed, this became more frequent. Since Gus was a rather impatient man, he would often get angry with himself or with the communicative situation. When the anger occurred, his impatience with himself would increase, and he would try to *force* himself to complete the thought as fast as he could. If he stumbled on a sound or word, he would try to say the word over and over, each time getting more frustrated and anxious. As this would happen, the speech disruptions would increase, and so would the anomic blocks or temporary losses of the ability to formulate the thought or word.

Over time, Gus developed the habit of looking to his wife to complete the thought for him, when all else failed and he could not recall the word. This worked for him. However, others would get anxious speaking with him as they empathized with him and began to experience the same feelings. They would watch him struggle and try to finish his thought for him, only realizing that what they thought he wanted to say was not right! With time, people started to avoid speaking with Gus, and he, too, started to avoid speaking opportunities. Imagine that amount of extra stress – for Gus, his wife, and others.

Stress should not be taking place within a communicative interchange. If it does, it will only play more havoc with self-expression in speech. When I was in training at the University of Miami Mailman Center for Child Development, which was a branch of the school of medicine, we as speech pathology trainees often had to present specific cases in an amphitheater filled with physicians. Being lowly students, and not having a whole lot of confidence, we frequently rambled and bumbled our way through a case presentation while simultaneously and profusely perspiring.

This same phenomenon may often occur for the person with mild aphasia. Because their ability to recall or formulate language is disrupted, especially under communicative, situational pressure, they may learn to fear speaking situations and withdraw quietly. Speaking, then, becomes more stressful, and actually may become somewhat painful. As speaking confidence diminishes, the person with the speaking difficulty may rely more upon their caregiver to help out in a speaking jam. With time, both speaker and caregiver anticipate speaking difficulty, and the caregiver takes on more of the speaking or *translating* responsibility.

We all know how habits are easily developed and how terribly difficult they are to break. Some interesting approaches I have used through the years, which are quite unlike many traditional approaches, were taken from *The School of Common Sense*, or *Hard Knocks University*. Many of the methods I have used are eclectic, but seem to work well. They were developed through much trial and error. Prior to presenting the methodology, I want you to look at some assumptions.

Review

1. Stress should be kept to a minimum when talking.
2. Do your best to keep the speaking opportunity relaxed.

Speech as an Unconscious Process

I believe speech is an automatic function. If you were to look at true elegance or competence in almost any human endeavor, you would see that it is a learned behavior that becomes automatic. When we look at true elegance or genius in any field, those who have reached that potential cannot always explain how they do what they do; they just do it! People reach a certain level of competence with practice, and then it gets integrated into the nervous system. If you look at dancers, singers, tennis players, physicians, surgeons, etc., there comes a time when all one really has to do is "show up" and the *genius* or the *competence* presents itself. I can attest to years and years of worrying what I would do with a patient when they showed up for the next appointment. There comes a time after one has practiced a specific discipline when you just *know* what to do.

It's like speaking. You get a phone call from a friend, a girlfriend, a son, daughter, or distant relative, and *you don't have to worry about what to say or how you will say it*, because that's the way it is when you have reached an unconscious level of competence. So, why am I having this conversation with you as a caregiver or speech-language pathologist? It is because I truly believe, from the depths of my clinical fiber, that when you are helping someone who has a "mild" expressive communication difficulty, you should not be overly concerned about training

135

them with conscious therapy "exercises." They already have the "knowledge" of speaking, but they do not always have *access* to the word or thought. It is a matter of *helping them gain access to the information*, not necessarily reteaching it or having them relearn it.

Please remember that true competence or elegance occurs subconsciously and automatically, which means that it comes without "trying." The elegant speech language pathologist or caregiver will do everything possible to facilitate that "automatic" speech, and often it comes with anger, delight, or excitement about a specific idea or topic, to which many of you will attest.

Create a Speaking Situation That Is as Natural as Possible

Therefore, in my approach to therapy, I want to create a speaking situation that is as *natural* as possible. Communication exchanges occur around things that the PCD is passionate or knowledgeable about, things he will want to talk about, and topics that he likes, appreciates, or enjoys. Conversations then ensue without fixating on errors or problematic features. We want to create conversation that is natural and *normal*, just as if the PCD were at home, or on the phone with their best friend or buddy. That is why, if one were to camp outside the door to my office, one would hear laughter, guffaws, and interactions as if best friends were meeting for the finest BS session of their lives. We want to get the PCD's attention away from their problem or speaking difficulty and focused on cool things to talk about. Now what does this approach do for the communicative interchange?

First, it gets the PCD's attention away from what is *wrong* with them. Most truly experienced clinicians who get results know that. Focusing on the problem or what is wrong usually invites further frustration and eventual clinical disaster. But more than that, getting the person to focus on expressing themselves about something they truly are interested in gets them *focused on that and NOT what is wrong with them*. There is a principle called *inhibition*, or *being inhibited*, which I believe occurs in cases of speaking or, for that matter, ANY behavior where an individual becomes overly concerned or worried about performance, which actually intensifies the harmful effects of such. There are many well-meaning clinicians who unfortunately focus there.

The trick is to find topics of interest that awaken the interest and desire to speak in the PCD. When that occurs, and the subject is of interest, the focus of attention is diverted to the matter at hand. When one talks about interest or passions, the feelings associated with those passions and interests emerge. Passions and interests tend to release inhibitions rather than facilitating them; likewise, focusing on inhibitions tends to keep them present. Allow the person with whom you are speaking to speak in a way that is not threatening or punishing. Sometimes you may want to model a slower speech rate for them so that it will give them more time to formulate what they wish to say. There are some cases in which you will not have to modify anything about how they are speaking; just concentrate solely on allowing the PCD to express themselves in an accepting environment, without correcting or castigating them.

The thought here is to get the person with the speaking difficulty to become more uninhibited, to forget the restraints that he or she or others have placed upon themselves or, for that matter, even to forget about the constraint of the stroke or head injury. This approach has been used by some experienced speech clinicians for years with speech handicapped persons, such as those with stuttering-like behaviors. You actually stimulate them to focus away from their preoccupation with self and their ways of speaking, and just have some fun talking about *cool stuff.*

Relax!

Getting back to Gus, when he and his wife first came in, they brought a shopping list of all his speaking problems! This was wrong and that was wrong, and he's saying "him" for "her" and "her" for "him" and gets his tenses mixed up, etc., and when am I going to work on that with him? I told both of them to "RELAX, and that would all be addressed in due time." I invited Gus and his wife to *chill,* and invited them to spend the visit with me getting to know one another. I found out that Gus and his wife and I had a passion for motorcycles, and listened non-stop as Gus told me about the trips they had taken in Texas, and some of their favorite restaurants and barbeque places. We talked about his love for never making a detailed plan of where they would be going on their trips, and how on the spur of the moment they would decide to take some road wherever it would lead them. You see, Gus was a totally uninhibited motorcycle rider when he and his wife would get on the bike or whenever they traveled. It often led them to places they had never thought of visiting.

It was amazing that, as I listened to Gus talk about their many travels, his speech was much more fluent, and there were fewer anomic errors or confusions. He rarely looked to his wife to supply him with a word or thought. He would periodically stop and point out that he did not think his speech was any better, and I would tell him to forget about what was wrong, and to tell me more about his travels! As he continued to share some of the wonderful tales of his life, there would be occasions of expressive difficulty. However, after two or three seconds of speaking confusion, I would invite him to say: "I'll think of it in a minute," and then forget about it and continue on in the conversation. He followed my instructions explicitly, and a surprising thing happened. He did not struggle at all, because he just moved on in the conversation if he got stuck. He did not have to sit there trying to grope or struggle for a word that was not there, and of course would not be there if he had any negative emotion.

Memory and language formulation just don't work well under duress! (And I must admit here there are some well-meaning family members and therapists who place their loved ones in stressful situations by paying too much attention to what they are doing wrong, rather than what they are doing right.) The wonderful thing is, when Gus says: "I'll think of it in a minute," it provides him an exit from a closed loop system that only invites stress and communicative breakdowns. It gives him an exit BEFORE the groping and STRUGGLE occur. But the best thing of all was that Gus would actually *recall* what it was that he could not say moments before, and typically be able to complete the thought later in the conversation. In addition, the negative feedback loop that he had always ended up with got bypassed, so that he didn't have to go down that same road of struggle, additional speech frustration and disruption. Gus has learned how to maintain composure.

The Power of the Pause

Another wonderful technique that worked for Gus and others like him utilized the *power of the pause*. Pause means to stop, and I like to teach others to pause with ease and grace. A pause is often a temporary stop caused by uncertainty, and I don't know about you, but for most people, it is difficult to proceed with anything which takes thought if there is uncertainty. Many of us have learned to wait until we are more certain before proceeding, including Gus, who used to barge through and struggle past the communicative block without fully knowing what to say, or how he would say it. Most normal talkers just proceed with talking, even when they are not sure of what they truly want to say. At times, that may result in a major communication error. What I like to teach those with mild speaking difficulties is to pause when the thought or word is NOT there. That PAUSE is an unconscious invitation to the person with whom he is speaking to take a turn. I believe it is also an *opportunity* to rest, *cool off the information processor, and give someone else an opportunity to speak.* It temporarily relieves the person of the stress from speaking and the ardent desire to be understood.

Whoa!

Speech rate is measured in words spoken per minute (WPM), and the speed a car travels is measured in miles per hour (MPH). Speech rate (WPM) is similar to miles per hour (MPH) since both deal with the speed of forward movement. Whether we are conversing about current events or jumping in the car, I look at both of these events synonymously.

So, let's think for a minute that we want to go for a drive in the car and wish to get to our destination in one hour. If we are familiar with the distance to our destination, know what road we will take and the speed limit for the road and the road conditions based on the time of day and day of the week, we can make a pretty close determination as to the time we will arrive. We realize that if the highways are relatively free from traffic, we can travel at approximately 65-70 miles per hour, and get to our destination in plenty of time. We know how fast we can travel on the roads we are taking, and have a pretty good idea of the traffic. We then tell the people at the destination what time we should arrive. We do not have to pull out calculators, road maps, or other measurement devices because we know subconsciously all the factors that go into the determination of approximate time of arrival; that is, if we are familiar with the route and destination. We just get in the car, start it, put it in gear, put on the iPhone, music, or news channel, and away we go. We can drink a coke and have a conversation with the wife about who was at the dinner party last night and what took place. Before you know it, you are at the destination without having to think about anything other than keeping your eyes open and scanning to the right, left and the road ahead. Speaking is very much like that.

However, let's say that you just had the car serviced and tires rotated and that they failed to balance one of the tires. You got out on the highway, and the steering wheel started to vibrate and shake. You are at the customary speed of 65 mph, and the whole front end of the car is shaking, plus there is a terrible vibration in the steering wheel. You decrease the speed of the car and, as you do, the car stops shaking at 50 mph. You try to accelerate again, and as the car reaches the speed of 65 MPH, it starts to shake and vibrate again. You decrease the forward speed of the car until it stops shaking, and now you are at 50 MPH once again. You stay at that speed until you reach the destination, because you know that if you speed up, the car will shake uncontrollably and become difficult to maneuver. Before you leave the destination for home, your mental computer has already figured that it will take another half hour or forty-five minutes to get home at 50 MPH, and you really haven't even thought about it very much, because you have subconsciously already realized that you will be driving home at a much slower speed and that it will take considerably longer to get there.

This description of the car and destination is what I believe happens with people who have brain injury and difficulty maintaining fluent speech. Like the car that cannot maintain the standard speed of 65-70 MPH on the highway due to a missing or malfunctioning part, a brain with a malfunctioning part cannot produce fluent speaking at the individual's habitual speech rate. Therefore, speech goes out of control with anomia or loss of words, language formulation difficulties and, in some cases, trouble comprehending spoken language. However, like the car, when the speed of forward movement is decreased, speech is more readily comprehended and formulated by the speaker. Not only that, but many can express themselves more readily because the language processor in the brain, although damaged, can often handle the load of information at a slower speed.

In Gus's case, we did not have to alter speech rate, although in many who have mild aphasia and speech disruptions, a definite decrease in rate gives the individual more time to formulate language as it is spoken, in addition to increased use of the pause to give the brain an opportunity to "cool off," or to give the other person a turn at speaking.

No Self-Deprecating Comments or Excuses, Please

Another key intervention with people who have a mild expressive aphasia and difficulty speaking is to encourage them NOT to make self-deprecating comments or excuses about their speaking, or why they can't say this or that. Gus was his own worst critic. Whether you are a husband, wife, child, or co-worker, no one benefits from criticism, whether it is from yourself or an outside source. Criticism is very detrimental to the normal process of speaking, due to the upset it typically causes. Those who speak normally are often not self-judgmental, nor are they criticized for the way they speak. Criticism often leads to internal negative emotion on the part of the person who receives it, and should be discouraged at all costs, because it has a harmful effect on thought and speaking expression. In an article on stuttering and stammering by Morales, of the Speech Care Center, the author refers to many factors thus far covered in this text which deal with time pressures, rapid speech, pressures in communication, speaking demands, rate of speech, and the speaking environment. Morales also includes a form of neurogenic stuttering or speech disruptions, that displays hesitancies, speech blocks, and difficulty uttering some words and phrases due to brain damage, traumatic head injury, or stroke.

> *Parents are in a key position to manipulate the child's environment to help their child recover. Time pressure is difficult for children who stutter. Examples of this pressure include: a rapid-paced lifestyle, wherein family members speak rapidly or interrupt each other; rapid-fire questions addressed to the child; reduced time in turn taking in conversation, etc. Other pressures in communicating include demand speech (i.e. parental requests for speech performance/recitation, translation for family members who don't speak English, parents' demands for a verbal explanation which may be emotionally and/or linguistically difficult for the child, etc.). Reducing time pressure, increasing time for taking turns in conversation, reducing demands upon the child to speak, and decreasing the rate of speech addressed to the child are helpful ways to manipulate the child's environment.[27]*

Many of the same concerns and approaches are used with stroke patients today who have developed speaking blocks that are referred to above as a neurogenic stutter. Neurogenic stuttering is a type of fluency disorder in which a person has difficulty in producing speech in a normal, smooth fashion. Individuals with fluency disorders may have speech that sounds fragmented or halting, with frequent interruptions and difficulty producing words without effort or struggle. Neurogenic stuttering typically appears following injury or disease to the central nervous system; i.e., the brain and spinal cord, including cortex, subcortex, cerebellar, and even the neural pathway regions. These injuries or diseases include:

- Cerebrovascular accident (stroke), with or without aphasia
- Head trauma
- Ischemic attacks (temporary obstruction of blood flow in the brain)
- Tumors, cysts, and other neoplasms/growths

---

27   Sarah Morales, BS, "Stuttering or Stammering," Children's Speech Care Center; A Division of Lynne Alba Speech Therapy, Professional Corporation, Accessed September 2011, http://www.childspeech. net/u_iv_l.html.

- Degenerative diseases, such as Parkinson's disease or Multiple Sclerosis (MS)
- Other diseases, such as meningitis, Guillain-Barré Syndrome, and AIDS
- Drug-related causes from medications"

Gus learned to pause and just be silent when he found it difficult to speak, which gave him a moment to relax and get curious about what he wanted to say. This would frequently allow him some time to remain calm. If the word came to him, great; if not, he would politely say, "It'll come to me in a minute." He could then remain silent or even pose a question to the listener. If he chose to remain silent, as previously stated, it would be a cue to the listener to pick up on the conversation, or "take a turn."

You Don't Go Back

Another wonderful strategy for working with mild expressive speaking difficulties is a rule I learned as an actor in the theatre that helps disguise the speaking problem. In my many years of working with mildly aphasic patients and mild stuttering, I found it very beneficial to teach my PCD's this simple rule of speaking: *Once you have said what you said, continue with the utterance, rather than going back and repeating any previous word(s) before it.*

People who have mild aphasia or dysfluencies caused by neurogenic factors may start a phrase or sentence, pause, and say the phrase again and again until they get unstuck. Trying to force through an utterance by repeating it over and over is rarely successful. I once had a PCD who would repeat the same phrase more than five or six times, and still not complete it.

Example

"I was going to tell you about my uh, uh, uh........darn.......I don't think I can say it.....

I was going to tell you about my uh, uh.....my.....uh....you know....... I just can't......

My uh........friend........uh......yeah...........my...... uh friend.........who.....uh.....I don't know why this keeps happening.....my friend...........I was going to tell you about........."

This example shows you explicitly how a PCD can dig a hole for themselves by going on and on in a continuous loop of uncertain and incomplete utterances. In this case, the person was instructed in the rule of what I call *You Don't Go Back*, the idea that once an utterance is stated, you can PAUSE, and *then complete the thought*. If one cannot complete the thought, one can say. "I'll think of it in a minute," ask a question to the listener, or just pause until the listener picks up on the nonverbal cue to continue the conversation. The key point in this intervention is not to repeat words or phrases said previously. To do so calls undue attention by the listener to the *way* one is speaking, rather than to the *content*. Dr. Van Riper would term this as a speaking difficulty worthy of therapy.

Example

Example of *You Don't Go Back* procedure with practice; same person as above example following training:

"I was going to tell you about my uh..........friend......

who I...............went to school with. Jared......was his name.....

He's...................dead now."

Review

1. Help the PCD get access to words and thoughts by stimulating speech on subjects of high interest or value.
2. Keep conversation stimulated on enjoyable subjects and experiences, not what is wrong with their speaking.
3. Automatic speech does NOT occur when "trying."
4. Uninhibited speaking occurs when no thought of what is "wrong" occurs, and the focus is on the conversational topic.
5. When a speech block occurs, pause.
6. Decreasing speech rate often allows the speech and language processor more time to formulate language and improves motor performance in speaking.
7. No self-deprecating comments, Please.
8. Once you have said what you said, continue speaking and move forward; don't go back and repeat any previous words or phrases.

The Cure Versus
Compensation and Adaptation

I love working with people who have speaking difficulties. Many of them are predictable, as I would be also if I were in their shoes. One of the comments frequently heard during the early sessions of therapy is: "I want to be the way I was before; I want to talk like I did, and walk and think like I did before. That's my goal, to be the way I was before."

When I hear someone tell me this, there is a mild sinking feeling that goes through my body. After working with thousands of patients, and watching what happens with them over time, I am convinced that many will make significant strides and improvements, but few ever return to pre-stroke or pre-neurogenic disease levels.

I believe that we, as therapists and caregivers, need to be realistic about finding the "cure," or stating what may likely occur in the future.

I believe we must tell the people we are working with that we will help them recover as much of their speaking and communication as possible. We are not crystal ball readers and cannot predict the extent of the speaking function's return. We must tell them the truth, and inform them that we will teach them how to compensate as much as possible for their speaking difficulty. We rarely find a cure, but we will help them speak as normally as

144

they can. That will be contingent on the methods we use, and their response to stimulation.

I personally believe that the speech-language pathologist and caregiver do help the PCD learn how to compensate for their speaking difficulty. We teach them to speak slower, use pauses, and give them a host of other methods as a way of *adapting* and *compensating*, so they can use what they now have in terms of function, and use it in the best way possible — and that's what I think we do as professionals and caregivers in the area of communication with our PCDs and loved ones. What I tell a patient is this: "I will do my very best to help you improve your speaking to the best of your ability." It is rare for anyone to take exception to that statement.

Review

We rarely help the person with the speaking difficulty return to "exactly the way they were before." Rather, we help each person adapt or compensate to improve their speaking condition to the best of their ability.

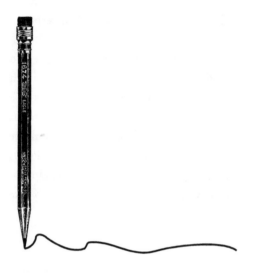

Conclusion

There may be some concepts presented in this book that seem foreign, but they will make sense as you practice them. I will now summarize some of the basic fundamentals that have been presented. Please go back and review any of these principles. An online webinar will be periodically launched that will demonstrate all of the procedures set forth in *The Teaching of Talking*, so that you can watch and listen to how the method is practiced. This will facilitate more rapid learning of the procedures, thereby enabling you and the person you are working with to be successful with the teaching and with the improvement of talking.

Sign up at www.teachingoftalking.com to be notified when we launch our new online instructional program. It will review the fundamentals of this text and demonstrate our instructional methods from the Embedded Question to the "I'll tell you about me if you tell me about you."

As I conclude the writing of this text, I think about the core principles and values that I live by in clinical practice.

Assessment

You must have an understanding of what the PCD is presenting when they attempt to speak. Please make sure that you take the time to *observe* and note what is *different* about the individual with whom you are speaking — and when I say *different,* I mean what it is that makes this individual and the act of speaking *different* from the norm. In his book, *Speech Correction, Principles and Methods,* Dr. Charles Van Riper states that: "Speech is abnormal when it deviates so far from the speech of other people that it calls attention to itself, interferes with communication, or causes the speaker or his listeners to be distressed."[28]

With practice, you may get very good at doing *speech screenings* each time you enter into a conversation with anyone (like it or not), at work or at play. You may get to the point where you will have your "clinical ears on" wherever you may be. On most days, I have conversations with many people. However, if there is anything *different* about anyone's speech, my eyes and ears totally focus to see, hear, and feel what is happening, and for a moment, *I internally model what it is they are doing with their speaking.* In a way, I actually become that person and model exactly what they are doing in my imagination. I experience firsthand what they are doing.

Once I have done this, I begin to model what I would do with my own speech if I were speaking that way. Then I show the PCD the "updated, corrected model," which is at a level of difficulty that I believe they can accomplish based upon my observations of their speaking. The model that I give them has already been practiced inside my head to see if they can duplicate it. In most cases they can, with a positive degree of accuracy. If they cannot, I start to test more deeply the areas that they were not able to do. Areas to be tested are those that are readily demonstrated by the PCD, which might include further tests of recall, articulation, speech rate, prosody, latency, vocal range, respiratory support, etc. By testing, you can find out how accurately the PCD can duplicate the way you speak if you show him with specific methods (stimulability testing). By doing this, you can see what the speech mechanism and the individual can tolerate. You basically test *tolerances* and find out what to address first; what I like to call finding the "best bang for the buck." What is the first alteration in the speaking process that will make the biggest contribution to speech intelligibility, or diminish the "weird" way they talk?

The other day, I saw a patient who said to me, "My speech sounds *retarded* and I hate that!" Immediately, I knew what he was talking about. He had a

---

28   VanRiper, Speech Correction Principles and Method,s 6ᵗʰ ed.(1978),p.43.

dysarthria, or slurred speech. I told him: "Let's see how we can diminish your speech sounding so *retarded*." I got his attention *–I stepped into his model of the world and acknowledged what he told me about his speech (that it sounded retarded) –* and then he was willing to do whatever was necessary. We increased the latency of time between each word spoken in the sentence and kept the vocal pitch within a very restricted range, as compared to the habitual and variable range of pitch that was initially presented. He was happy to be shown how to improve his speech by being presented a model of how I knew it *could sound*. The intelligibility in tests of stimulability went from 33% to over 80%, and this was only during the evaluative session! Remember that a test of stimulability is intended to show the PCD a model of how their speech *could* sound, and seeing and hearing if they can duplicate it.

Rapport

Establishing rapport is critical for a successful outcome. You want to *connect* with each and every person who shows up at your office door. You must be able to identify what their speaking difficulty is and how you are going to correct it. That is why I model it in my mind or out loud as the PCD is sitting across from me. Modeling the problem should give you a good idea of how it is going to be remediated or, pardon the expression, how it is going to be *fixed!* Before that person leaves the office, he or she should know whether speech therapy will be helpful or not.

We can address almost any speaking concern during the evaluation visit and demonstrate how it can be improved upon. After thoroughly testing the act of speaking, we identify the difficulty and model a better way to say it. The presentation is plain and simple, so the PCD can experience improved speaking within just a few minutes. They leave the evaluation visit excited and hopeful, knowing that they came to the right place and person. With hope for the improvement of talking, they are excited about the prospect of therapy, expecting an answer and anticipating improvement. You have connected with them because you addressed the problem they came with and demonstrated the probability of improvement. If you can do that, they will not only be excited about the possibility of achieving what they came to you for, but they will immediately like and respect you for addressing their concerns and showing them with honesty and integrity what they can expect from therapy.

In the previous example of the patient who came in and said, "My speech sounds retarded and I hate that," I went to what we call his "model of the world."

This is a concept from Neuro-Linguistic Programming (NLP)©[29] whereby the clinician (or anyone who has this knowledge) identifies the individual's belief system by listening to their expressive language. What we say aloud is often a self-fulfilling prophesy. In this example, the PCD is telling us that he thinks his speech sounds "retarded." That is his belief. No matter what we say to him, we *all* know that it does sound *retarded*; either that or it sounds like he just drank a fifth of Jack Daniels! By agreeing with him and saying "*You are right, it does sound retarded and we are going to see right now how to make your speech more natural,*" he realizes immediately that because we entered into his model of the world, no one is going to discount what he is saying; in fact, we are actually agreeing with him. When one has agreement, the relationship can move forward. We know from our own experiences in life that when there is *no agreement*, relationships rarely develop or last.

Too often, people come in for evaluations and examinations and leave with no clue as to whether they have a problem that would be amenable to therapy. It is my sincere belief that a person who has taken the time and expense to have an evaluation should be offered an explanation and a relative idea regarding goals and the prognosis for improvement. It is only courteous, whenever possible, to provide that.

Fun and Humor

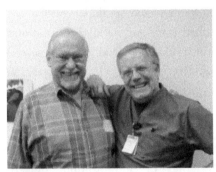

Fun and humor are on the hit parade of what I value during any clinical visit. If you can wake up each and every morning excited about who you will be seeing and what you will be doing that day, then you could practice this profession for decades. Practicing speech language pathology, for me, is like having seven or eight of my best friends stop by for a chat two or three times a week, and the amazing thing is that we get the results we want without a lot of frustration or angst. What we also get is fun, laughter, and achievement. It can be readily demonstrated that if a PCD is

29   NLP models patterns of human excellence. This includes the way people of excellence take in
     information from the world, how they describe it to themselves with their senses, filter it with their
     beliefs and values, and act on the result, *http://www.inspiritive.com.au/glossary.htm*.

relaxed and there is humor and laughing, they cannot be thinking of doom and gloom at the same time.

Therapy should also be covert. By that, I mean that whenever possible, you should work on their goals without necessarily having them "try." Often, the more a person tries, the more failure and frustration there is. This is not the fault of the PCD, but rather of the clinician: either the task is too difficult or too much undue attention is paid to the problem (*what's wrong*) rather than the solution. Recently, I was seeing a person with an *apprehension about speaking* with friends and family. Over time, the PCD *had come to expect failure when speaking*, and therefore the expectation was realized. What we expect usually happens.

We did not even address the "problem" of stuttering. We just talked about *being relaxed, speaking slowly* and *taking as much time as he wanted to say what he wanted*. We started talking about his new car, house and funny neighbors. He learned how to pause the forward movement of speaking when a speech block occurred and to allow the other person to speak at that moment, therefore preventing a dysfluency of speech. We had conversations about his dog, his wife, and the challenges following his stroke. We laughed and giggled about the funny things that happen in life and how to look at speaking and the behaviors associated with it in a much lighter, more humorous way. We laughed and cut up all through the visit; and the funny thing was that the more we laughed and found humor in what we were doing, the more fluent his speech became. No dread, no doom, no fear — none of the things that make speaking worse.

An interesting phenomenon that resulted from our weekly conversational sessions was that he was no longer fearful of speaking. He had plenty of success speaking comfortably in therapy and was able to carry that feeling of success out of the therapy room into his world.

Making it Easy

When I was younger, my parents wondered why I was not an achiever like my twin brother and sister. It seemed as if they always caught on to things quickly. Whenever they attempted to teach me anything, such as how to play a game or tie my shoes, it was always *failure*. They would say, "All you have to do is this and this, and then do this and that." By that time, I would have a blank stare on my face. They just didn't have a clue about how to present information to me so that I would get it. After a while they thought I was just a "dummy," and ceased asking me to play with them. I think something like that occurs with people who have lost the ability to speak, or those who have not yet learned it.

The distinction about this concept of *making it easy* is profound, and will be another foundation block in your approach to doing treatment with *The Teaching of Talking*. I thought for years and years that I was a dummy. That is what was drilled into my head over and over again by well-meaning family members who really *had no clue* about how to teach me so that I would *get it!* I thought I would never learn to tie my shoes or play gin rummy, cribbage, scrabble, or monopoly.

Then one day we had a babysitter by the name of Mrs. Myers, a gentle woman with whom I was instantly comfortable. I knew from the start that she would not tell me how stupid or wrong I was. The first thing this wonderful human being taught me was how to tie my shoes — ugh. So often, my brother and sister would do the same thing — show me real fast, say it real fast, and leave me scratching my head and trying to remember. Mrs. Myers was different. She broke up the task of tying shoes into five or six steps and made sure that I mastered each step in succession before progressing on to the next.

And that is the way we should do therapy. When it is done in a thoughtful, sequential manner, it can be fun and easy. First, I learned to pick up the ends of each shoelace and hold them out to the side. When I could do that consistently, she showed me how to cross the strings and then lay the ends down flat across the top of the shoe. When I could do the first two steps, she showed me how to lift the laces, take the right lace and pass it around and under the left one. It was this progression and then going back through each sequence before going to the next one that enabled me to learn how to tie my shoes in next to no time.

I thought I was just dumb and could never learn how to do anything like the other kids. *Wrong!* There are many people with speaking problems who are similar, and have not had the experience of working with an elegant therapist who can take almost any desired behavior and break it down into what I have coined, *"Tying Your Shoes Steps."*

Once Mrs. Myers showed me how to tie my shoes, I was eager at every opportunity to take off my shoes, put them back on, and re-tie them. I also regularly volunteered to tie my brother's and sister's shoes.

We practice this same principle in *The Teaching of Talking*. Once the PCD has the strategy partially learned for what to do in order to master a specific speech behavior, it must be practiced over and over again. My old friend, Dr. Gregory Cheatwood, used to repeat many times during his seminars that "repetition is the mother of all skill." With that in mind, as soon as I can get the PCD to do the desired behavior in single word speech, or phrases, I immediately attempt, just as soon as possible, to develop a *stimulated conversation* that is tailored and appropriate to the PCD's level of speaking difficulty. I want success, always, and that is why we strive to present models for the PCDs that we know instinctually will be readily spoken.

A stimulated conversation is initiated by the SM to determine whether the PCD can use the newly desired speaking behavior during discussion of a topic of interest. It can be stimulated with *Embedded Questions* and *Tell Me Phrases* — it does not have to be spontaneous. In fact, you can have a conversation and use *Embedded Questions* for most of it. Now, I think of astronauts in flight simulators. Stimulating conversation and sentences in the PCD is very much like the use of flight simulators by astronauts: the practice should be as much like the real thing as possible in order to prepare the user to think and react as they would in the real-life event.

If the PCD is not ready for a conversation, then we may practice single words or word pairs that are generated between the two of us during a conversation. The practice of space flight in simulation is like the practice of words, phrases or single sentences until the accuracy is at or near 100%. At that time, we work towards the expression of two-word combinations or more without any error, and then gradually increase the number of words, phrases, or sentences, until conversations take place.

While the astronaut works towards a very complex set of behaviors to operate a space craft, we and our PCD work toward the automaticity of expressive speech. For the PCD, *speech simulation* may be every bit as challenging as training to be an astronaut and taking countless hours of training in the flight simulator. Do you get it? When the PCD can have a conversation about any topic and successfully master the specific behavior, then you have "carry-over," or learning that has taken place at an automatic or unconscious level. That is the purpose of what we do as speech-language pathologists and SMs. Our sole purpose is to get the people we are working with to master a speaking behavior at an unconscious level so that it comes out of their mouths automatically.

Be an Exceptional Model

If you intend to be successful in your endeavors as a speech-language pathologist, caregiver, loved one, or SM, you must be able to model for the individual exactly what you expect from them in terms of their speaking. Often the family member or caregiver expects the person with the speaking difficulty to know what they should do as compared to what they are actually doing. *Wrong!* So often I have heard well-meaning family members or caregivers say:

"If you would just slow down or talk like you used to, you wouldn't be in this mess. That was how my parents and siblings talked to me about tying shoes!" *But I didn't know what to do any more than the PCD does when he or she shows up at your door!*

You must model exactly what you want them to sound like, and make it simple enough so that they can model it readily. It is at this point where you begin to *test the tolerances* of the person and their speaking mechanism to see whether you should be at the single word, phrase, or sentence level. You will know exactly at what level you need to be by finding out exactly what they CAN DO when you give them the new model. Make sure that you give them a task they can be successful at. That is where you start, and then make the task gradually more difficult, only proceeding when they are again successful.

Make sure your voice is loud enough, your articulation is accurate, your speed is slow, and the task is easy enough. In the last year I have given seminars on *The Teaching of Talking*, where I have met some very interesting speech-language pathologists and caregivers. I was delighted to meet some who were exceptional SMs, with impeccable speech, voice, loudness, and rate of speaking. However, I also met some who spoke so fast that I could hardly follow what they were saying. There were others who had weak voices or imprecise articulation. Ask yourself this question in regard to your way of speaking. Is there anything about your speech that could get in the way of being an exceptional SM? (See Self Evaluation Form on page 41 or online at www.teachingoftalking.com) These very simple forms may give you some valuable feedback that, perhaps, you had not considered previously. If there is anything you question about your personal speaking ability, it would be good to fill out this form, and to have at least three people you admire and respect fill one out for you as well.

Never Make Anyone "Wrong"

One of the ways to throw a monkey wrench into the gears of your professional or personal relationships is to let other people know how wrong they are. That is the road to failure in any relationship. Remember this: *No one likes to be told they are wrong* — not your kids, your wife, your spouse, your mother or father, or even the garbage man! Therefore, if you will adopt this approach to humanity, it will go better for you in the overall scheme of things. Of course, the people you work with in the stimulation of speech and language do not want to be told they are wrong either. One of the reasons they will have chosen you to be the model for their speech is out of trust that you will not make them "wrong."

Here is a clean-cut rule. If you will adopt it, things will go better with the person you are helping; in fact, they will go better in *any* interpersonal relationship. In therapy, when the person with whom you are working makes an error or does not say what you are working on correctly: *Restimulate! Restimulate! Restimulate! Restimulate!*

Restimulation is a very simple concept, its intention being to provide the model more clearly and succinctly again for the PCD. It's not about saying "No," or "You screwed up again." It is about saying, "Let's do that again. Can you say: 'Let's ➔ go ➔ home'?", or "That was close. I am going to say it again for you: 'Let's ➔ Go ➔ HOME!' Now, you say: 'LET'S GO HOME!'"

So, the rule of thumb here is: When you don't get the response you want, provide the model for them again, possibly slower, perhaps emphasizing the syllables or changing your loudness or tonality. When they don't get it, take on the responsibility that it is *you* who has to *change the model.*

Share Who You Are as a Human Being with Others

Years ago, at the start of my career, I enrolled in "How to Win Friends and Influence People," offered by the Dale Carnegie organization. It introduced tried and true suggestions for developing and maintaining personal relationships. In fact, it was one of the best "continuing education courses" I have ever taken.

I learned through the Dale Carnegie coursework that people are more comfortable if you allow them to know who *you* are, sharing similar concerns and frailties. They will appreciate that you are genuine, not just a professional *know it all!* Once rapport has been established, they will open up and share who *they* are, and the challenges they face.

Be More and Do More Than they Expect

If you have read any self-development books, this credo will be repeated over and over again. It is really nothing new. However, it is worthy of adoption into the way we practice and interact with the people who need our services. It does not matter if you are a spouse, a caregiver, or a speech-language pathologist. Do your best, and do more than anyone expects. Give more than they expect. Promise more than you would expect from yourself, and fulfill whatever you have promised. When the PCDs make statements of opinion or hope, acknowledge those statements and do whatever you can to satisfy that hope.

There was a person who came to Houston for therapy from out west, and he was going to be here for a short period of time. The therapist who evaluated this PCD suggested the "status quo" frequency of three therapy sessions weekly. The person's wife said: "Gee whiz, I wish we could be seen more often since we will only be here for a short period of time, about a month." Does it sound reasonable to you that the wife of a person who needed speech therapy, in town at a hotel for a month, should make a request for more therapy? You betcha! The task, then, is for you to do whatever is humanly possible to be an advocate for that person and get the therapy that you believe would be beneficial for them. Do more than you would typically do, and deliver everything you say you are going to do.

One of my professors, early in my training at the University of Miami, once told me to "treat each PCD as if they were a best friend, family member or relative." After that suggestion, I would go way beyond what was "standard" in the attention and treatment of those persons because I saw each and every one of them as members of my family.

And finally, if you love *all* people with *all* of your heart and soul, you will love almost everyone; even those you don't like. I challenge you to love more, give more, and your life will overflow with more happiness, goodness and well-being.

*Farewell, Shalom, Salem, Adios, Arrivederci, Sayonara

Peace and Love to You and Yours,

Mark A. Ittleman, M.S., CCC/SLP
Houston, Texas
December, 2011

*Used as a traditional greeting or farewell. These words may also signify welfare of every kind: security, contentment, sound health, prosperity, friendship, peace of mind and heart, as opposed to dissatisfaction and unrest.

The Good Life

To laugh often and much;
To win the respect of intelligent people
and the affection of children;
To earn the appreciation of honest critics
and endure the betrayal of false friends;
To appreciate beauty, to find the best in others;
To leave the world a bit better, whether
by a healthy child, a garden patch
or a redeemed social condition;
To know even one life has breathed
easier because you have lived.
This is to have succeeded.[30]

The Five Most Important Things in Life

If any of us were to list the five most
important things in life; what would they be?

A sense of meaning.
A feeling of personal fulfillment.
Having people who really care about us.
Having basic necessities—food, shelter, health.
And contentment and peace.[31]

---

30   -- "Widely attributed to Emerson on the internet, this actually originates with "What is Success?" by
Bessie Anderson Stanley, in Heart Throbs, Volume Two (1911), Edited by Joseph Mitchell Chapple.
The "Good Life," Happiness: Eudaimonia; thoughts from different traditions; http//doggo.tripod.
com/dogggoodlife.html.

31   Merle Good and Phyllis Pellman Good, "The Amish," 20 Most Asked Questions About the Amish &
Mennonites, rev. ed. (1995; repr., Intercourse, PA 17534: Good Books, 1979), 20.

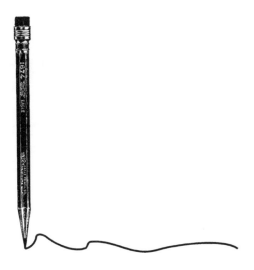

Epilogue

I have caught the spirit of people who have gone down in history for making a major contribution to humanity. Some of my favorite people are Napoleon Hill, Charles Lindbergh, Thomas Alva Edison, Amelia Earhart, Dr. Milton Erickson, and more recent travelers, Tony Robbins, Brendon Buchard, and Steve Jobs. I feel as though I know them intimately. We are kindred spirits through a commitment to life dreams. Something magical happens when you are able to live your dream. I have been thinking it, doing it, creating it, committing to it, talking about it, and on the playing field with it, each and every day for more hours than I ever thought possible. When that happens, there is a sixth sense that others have described, a knowing and a wisdom that are transmitted to the mind of the individual with that commitment.

So I challenge you, dear reader, as I did at the beginning: Pursue your life dreams! I hope that this brief ride on my bus has given you a glimpse into the joy and excitement you can experience when you learn to stimulate speech and language in those who need you. The teaching of talking is *not* a "job" or a "career"! It is a way of life, a part of your innermost being, the definition of *who* you are, and your *major* contribution to humanity.

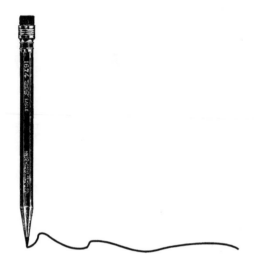

About the Author

Mark A. Ittleman, M.S., CCC/SLP, is a speech-language pathologist whose patients have called him *"the speech pathologist who can make a rock talk!"* He has practiced the "art" of speech therapy for forty years and is a true expert.

Mark was the founding speech-language pathologist of a residential program for aphasic patients, and has conducted research to find the best methods for training others to talk. He is a much-sought-after speaker due to his enthusiasm and commitment to teaching others a new and nontraditional way of practicing speech therapy.

Besides being an expert speech-language pathologist, he is a gifted author, seminar leader, mentor, and teacher of speech-language pathologists and therapists. He also trains family members to be exceptionally good speech models (SMs) for those who have lost the ability to speak, in a way that is very similar to how children learn to talk: through interaction with loved ones at home.

Families love working with Mark, because his methods are non-confrontational and fun. His patients and clients appreciate his caring attitude and the humor that is always interspersed in therapy or training. People are amazed at his methods, which involve talking during the process of building/ rebuilding speech.

Ittleman is a member of the American Speech-Language and Hearing Association, holds the Certificate of Clinical Competence in Speech-Language Pathology, and is also a member of the Texas Speech-Language and Hearing Association. He is licensed as a speech-language pathologist. He is currently a Senior Speech-Language Pathologist at The Institute for Rehabilitation and Research (TIRR) at Memorial Hermann Hospital in Houston, Texas, which is world-famous for exceptional physical, occupational, and speech therapy. He will soon complete work there in pursuit of his dream of instructing others in *The Teaching of Talking* throughout the United States and the world. He will also publish additional works in speech language pathology for speech-language pathologists, caregivers, students, and health care professionals.

Glossary of Terms

A

Abnormal speech. Speech is abnormal when it is so different from the speech of others that it calls attention to itself, interferes with communication, or causes the speaker or his listeners to be distressed.

Activities of daily living (ADL). Activities that take place every day of one's life, often related to activities such as toileting, bathing, personal hygiene, dressing, eating, and cleaning up.

Adapting. Adapting or conforming oneself to new or different conditions.

Affricates. A stop (t) that is immediately followed by a fricative sound (sh) as in "(ch)" or "(j)" as the starting sound of a word.

Alternate Choice Question. A method used in *The Teaching of Talking* approach by which a question is posed that has words, syntax, and grammar within its structure to help the PCD formulate a single word, phrase, or sentence. However, the person with the communication difficulty (PCD) is given a choice within the question (now/later; hamburger/hot dog) which requires both thought and the ability to choose an answer. The reply is expressed by the PCD at the appropriate level of difficulty.

Am/Am Not Phrases. Of the phrase *to be*. PCD learns the use of "I am" in the present tense affirmative (I am thirsty/a man), and also learns it in the negative (I am not thirsty/a man.)

Anomic aphasia. An impaired ability to name objects, or to recognize written or spoken names of objects. An individual with anomic aphasia has word-finding difficulties. This is called anomia. The PCD struggles, and may be unable to find the right words for speaking and writing. There are various levels of severity.

Aphasia. A medical condition caused by brain trauma, injury, or disease, which reduces the ability to understand or express spoken and written language.

161

Apraxia (of speech). The inability to voluntarily produce or imitate vowels, speech sounds, words, or word combinations. Varies from mild to profound in severity.

Articulation. The ability to accurately formulate and express the specific speech sounds of a given language. Formulation requires fine coordination of the tongue, lips, teeth, and palate.

Auditory bombardment. Having the PCD *hear* sounds, words, phrases or sentences said repeatedly by a speech model. This is necessary in order for the PCD to accurately imitate what is heard.

Articulatory phonetics. The study of the production of speech sounds by the articulatory and vocal tract of the speaker.

B

Blend. A combination of two consonant sounds before a vowel, such as in the word "blame."

Broca's aphasia. A condition characterized by either partial or total loss of the ability to express oneself, either through speech or writing. Comprehension of what is heard is usually not affected. This condition may result from a stroke, head injury, brain tumor, or infection.

C

Calibration. The observation of body movements to determine the PCD's standard nonverbal responses to "yes" and "no"" questions.

Carry-over. The practice of any speaking behavior that, with repetition, becomes automatic.

Cerebellar. Pertaining to the cerebellum, the part of the brain in the back of the head between the cerebrum and the brain stem. The cerebellum controls balance for walking, standing and other complex motor functions, including motor speech. Often associated with dysarthria, or the slurring of speech.

Cerebrovascular accident. This results in stroke, the rapid loss of brain function(s) due to disturbance in the blood supply to the brain, such as in the case of ischemia (lack of blood flow) caused by blockage (thrombosis, arterial embolism), or of a hemorrhage (leakage of blood). As a result, the affected area of the brain cannot function, which may result in an inability to move one or more limbs on one side of the body, inability to understand or formulate speech, or an inability to see one side of the visual field.

Chunk. The number of words that a PCD can imitate in one utterance following a verbal example by the SM. The number of words within the chunk is dependent upon the immediate memory of the PCD. The length of the chunk should increase as speech is stimulated by the SM.

Circumlocutions. The subconscious or learned use of pantomime, nonverbal communication, or word substitution by a PCD because of recall difficulty.

Closet of life. PCDs may refuse to see friends and decline social opportunities. They may refuse to answer the phone, go to church, or participate in family events; they may withdraw, or avoid social and verbal interaction. Common in both children and adults.

CNA. Certified Nursing Assistant.

Communication sphere of consciousness. It really does not matter what or how something is being said, but rather that the speech model (SM) and person with the speaking difficulty (PCD) are expressing themselves in whatever way works, and that the conversation has life and purpose. What is important is that information is being shared and conveyed.

Compensating. To adjust (someone or something, especially oneself) to different conditions, a new environment.

Consciousness. A particular level of awareness and of paying attention, either internally within oneself or externally to what is happening in the environment.-

Consonant-Vowel Cluster. The combination of a consonant and a vowel when heard, seen, or said (ba, da, mo, ro, etc.).

Constraint Induced Language Therapy. A pragmatic form of speech and language stimulation that focuses on required speaking and the necessity for numerous repetitions to facilitate learning.

Cortex. The outer portion of the cerebrum.

Courtesy. Polite behavior that shows respect for people in social situations.

Covert. Made, shown, or done in a way that is not easily seen or noticed; secret or hidden.

Critic. A person who judges, evaluates, or criticizes; a fault finder.

D

Dancing in the conversation. Being so engaged in a conversation that you lose track of time.

Distributed practice. The process of learning with repeated trials over a specific period of time; i.e., speech therapy given three times a week on Monday,

Wednesday and Friday for twelve weeks, versus massed practice of training during a single unit of time.

Duress. Forcible restraint or restriction; compulsion by threat.

Dysarthria. Impaired articulatory ability resulting from defects in the peripheral motor nerves and muscle weakness of the structures in the speech mechanism; a general slurring of speech.

Dysfluencies. Interruptions in the smooth flow of speech, as by a pause or the repetition of a sound, syllable, word or phrase.

E

Embedded Questions. A method used in *The Teaching of Talking* approach by which a question is posed that has embedded within it the sounds, words, syntax, and grammar to help the PCD formulate a single word, phrase, or sentence. The embedded question is formulated in a *Yes/No* question by the SM, such as: SM: Do you like cake? PCD: Yes, I like cake.

Enrolling Conversations. Speaking from the heart in a way that is truly meant, in order to help someone move from a fixed position towards a new and often different objective or goal.

Evidence-Based Practice. Clinicians who base their treatment decisions on a balance of research-based evidence, clinical expertise and experience, and the client's wishes. It also includes the accurate reporting of progress based on observations and measurements.

Expressive language. The ability to speak and use written language to express oneself.

F

Focused auditory stimulation. Repeating and using your voice to model specific speech behaviors such as sounds, words, or ways of speaking in phrases or sentences. The words and manner of speaking are presented in such a way that they can be readily heard and imitated by the person with the communication difficulty.

Fricatives. A consonant speech sound such as (f), (v) or (sh), made by forcing an airstream through a constricted opening.

G

Generative stage. The stage at which the person with communication difficulty starts to use his own vocabulary and expressions in speaking.

Genius. Exceptional competence which comes from a commitment to a specific discipline.

H

Habitual speed. The speed at which one has always spoken.

Home program. A set of exercises or recommendations of what should be practiced at home, either during or at the completion of therapy.

I

"I'll tell you about me and you tell me about you" method. A method of speech therapy coined in *The Teaching of Talking* to stimulate expressive speech and language.

I'm/I am Phrases. Instruction in the grammar of *to be.*

Imitation. An act of copying someone's actions, words, or behavior.

Immediate memory. The ability to remember a small amount of information over a few seconds.

Independent language. The person with communication difficulty starts to use his own vocabulary and expressions spontaneously, or during language stimulation activities.

Informal testing. Observation of social interaction and communication between two or more people. Articulation, expressive language, voice, rate, resonance, and learning responses are observed and documented.

Inhibition. Something that forbids, debars, or restricts; an inner impediment to free activity, expression, or functioning, such as a mental process imposing restraint upon behavior or upon another mental process (such as a desire).

Inquiry. A question intended to obtain information about someone or something.

Ischemic attack. Temporary obstruction of the flow of blood in the brain.

J

Junkyard dog. A junk yard dog is trained to bite an intruder, and not to let go until his master gives him the command to "let go!" This concept in our text refers to *junkyard dog mentality, a persistent commitment to an endeavor, and never letting go or giving up until it is completed.*

L

Language. A shared system for communicating and exchanging knowledge, feelings, thoughts, and beliefs that involves sounds, signs, gestures, and/or spoken or written words.

Language samples. A language sample is a written record of the PCD's expressive speech and language. It is obtained by transcribing a recorded sample of everything said during the evaluation. The speech pathologist evaluates grammar, syntax or articulation using the language sample.

Latency. The amount of time between each spoken word within a phrase or sentence.

Lexicon. All of the words that one understands and expresses; vocabulary.

Lingua- alveolar. Pertaining to the tongue and how it contacts the roof of the mouth for the speech sounds (t), (d), (n), (l), (s), (sh), and (j).

Lingua-velar. Pertaining to sounds of speech that are produced with the tongue and the soft palate (k), (g).

Locatives. The distinctive function in language to indicate where something is located.

Long-term memory. The phase of the memory process considered to be the permanent storehouse of retained information.

M

Massed practice. Learning and practicing given behaviors over a single period of time.

Model of the world. The way one sees the world, and being cognizant and respectful of how others see and perceive it.

Motor bombardment. Repeating a given motor act, such as the repetition of a sound, word, phrase, or sentence many times, in order to facilitate motor learning of how something is said.

Motor programming. Repeated motor act that is done with frequency and intensity. This leads to improved motor memory for that specific movement. If I say "diadochokinesis," and have you repeat that word accurately a number of times, you will then have that word properly programmed motorically.

Motor Speech Disorders. Difficulty articulating speech due to a breakdown of electrical impulses coming from the nerves and muscles which are connected to the motor speech structures of the lips, teeth, tongue, and palate. Can lead to problems producing vowels, single syllables, words phrases and conversation accurately. Often due to weakness, or uncoordinated voluntary muscle movement.

Moto-kinesthetic. Physically moving any structure inside the mouth numerous times; i.e., the therapist can take hold of a person's tongue, move it to the left and right numerous times to retrain the tongue to move from left to right.

Multitasking. The performance of multiple tasks at one time.

N

Name recall. The ability to remember and express a name, word, or thought.

Native speakers (NS). The language one speaks from birth, usually pertaining to the place of birth.

Negative practice. Practicing or speaking in an incorrect way that further strengthens the negative speaking habit.

Neoplasms. New growths.

Neural pathway regions. Pathways and specific areas within the brain and nervous system that are responsible for specific functions, such as walking and talking.

Neurogenic stuttering. Speech disruptions including hesitancies, speech blocks, and difficulty uttering some words and phrases due to brain damage, traumatic head injury, and stroke.

Neuro-Linguistic Programming describes the fundamental dynamics between mind (neuro) and language (linguistic), and how their interplay affects our body and behavior (programming).

Nouns. Words that name a person, place, or thing.

O

Open-Ended Questions. An open-ended question is designed to encourage a full, meaningful answer using the subject's own knowledge and/or feelings. It is the opposite of a closed-ended question, which encourages a short or single-word answer. Open-ended questions also tend to be more objective and less leading than closed-ended questions. Open-ended questions typically begin with words such as "Why" and "How," or with phrases such as "Tell me about..." They are often not technically a question, but a statement that implicitly asks for a response.

P

Paraphasic. Unable to speak correctly, substituting one word for another, and jumbling words and sentences unintelligibly.

PCD. Person with Communication Difficulty. A person who has communication and/or speaking difficulties due to developmental, learning, or organic/neurological influences that affect how speech is produced with the lips, teeth, tongue, palate, and voice. A PCD may also have difficulty in the understanding or formation of language in reading, listening, writing or speaking.

Pedagogy. The methods and principles of teaching. The word comes from the Greek language and means "to lead the child." Referenced within *The Teaching of Talking* to compare to a caregiver, parent, or spouse.

Peripheral oral examination. This examination tests the structures of the speech mechanism, which include the lips, teeth, tongue, palate, and soft palate to see if they are functioning adequately for the production of speech. It is also a visual inspection of the speech mechanism and its structures to determine the presence of any physical abnormalities that could affect eating or speaking.

Phonemes. The smallest phonetic unit in a language that is capable of conveying a distinction in meaning, as the (m) of "mat" and the (b) of "bat" in English.

Phonetics. The study of the sounds used in speech.

Phrase Completion Method. A method to stimulate language wherein the SM says the start of a phrase and the person with communication difficulty completes it.

Physiology. In the context of *The Teaching of Talking*, the physical, nonverbal gestures and movements a person makes that helps the listener interpret what is being conveyed.

Placement and Manner. To place the mouth, tongue, and lips in the same position as the SM (***placement***), and to correctly imitate the movement and sound that is being presented by the speech model (***manner***).

Power of the pause. A temporary stop; a brief suspension of the voice to indicate the limits and relations of sentences and their parts; temporary inaction, used especially as a method within the *Teaching of Talking* to gather one's thoughts in order to complete a given thought.

Pragmatic. An approach that uses social interaction to improve the communication abilities of people with speaking difficulties. Teaching and requiring language at home during activities of daily living, where the PCD must ask for things or make requests to go places.

Predicate adjective. An adjective following a linking verb that describes the subject, such as "roses are red."

Predicate sequence. A complete thought (sentence) in speech, often comprised of the action of the subject, which is the predicate. In the sentence "John threw the ball," John is the subject and "threw the ball" is the predicate sequence.

Present in the conversation. Paying attention to the processes involved in conversation and to what the other person is saying, without being distracted by internal thoughts or dialogue.

Prognostic moment. The moment when a prediction for improvement of speech based on what is observed in the speaking of the PCD can be made. Usually occurs when new or unexpected speaking behaviors are observed.

Progressive verbs. Progressive tense verbs, which include present progressive, past progressive, future progressive, present perfect progressive, past perfect progressive, and future perfect progressive, describe a continuing action, and end in "-ing."

R

Rapport. A relationship in which people like, understand, and respect each other.

Reactive. Automatic response to an event instead of deliberate and purposeful (conscious) behavior.

Receptive language. The ability to comprehend language which is received via oral or written communication.

Recreating conversations. The ability of the listener or SM to clarify what was just spoken by the PCD. For example, "So I think what you are trying to tell me is that you would like to buy a new phone." This ensures that what was spoken is understood by the SM or listener.

Recreating a Conversation Method. A method of stimulating speech used in *The Teaching of Talking.*

Restimulation. When a PCD has difficulty responding, simply repeat the task.

S

"Say" Phrases. Words used by the SM to model words, phrases or sentences. The PCD is given the model of what to say, and is then stimulated to repeat or imitate what was said with urgency. For example, the SM says: "I WANT COFFEE." The PCD responds: "I want coffee." (Author's note: the voice should be used in such a way that the desired response is gotten immediately)

Self-fulfilling prophecy. A prediction that is often spoken or thought directly or indirectly by the SM or PCD. It can be negative or positive. Either way, it may actually become a reality if repeated often, leading to behaviors which take a person toward or away from a specific idea or goal. One of the goals of an elegant therapist is to repeat the desired outcome of the PCD, if attainable, so that the expectancy and achievement is anticipated and realized.

Semantic intent. Understanding the meaning of what was spoken or communicated by the individual.

Seven-repetition model. Repeating a stimulus word numerous times by having the PCD hear, see, or say it seven times.

Shadowing method. This method usually comes into play when the PCD has difficulty expressing a thought due to sound distortion in speaking, word choice, or order. The SM listens to the thought expressed, and first clarifies that he/she understood the PCD's intention. When clarified, the SM alters the utterance, and presents it back to the PCD in a different way to facilitate a more accurate and intelligible utterance. This can be done by modeling the words back to the PCD at a slower rate, or in simpler language.

Short-term memory. That section of the memory storage system of limited capacity (approximately seven items) that is capable of storing material for a brief period of time. Often used synonymously with ***immediate memory***. A popular example of short-term memory is the ability to remember a seven-digit telephone number just long enough to dial a call. In most cases, unless the number is consciously repeated several times, it will be forgotten.

Single-Word Level. A level of speaking ability where the PCD is stimulated to speak only single words, or one word at a time.

SLP. A Speech-Language Pathologist.

SM. A Speech Model. One who models and stimulates speech and language by using his/her voice, and speaks in such a way as to readily elicit speaking, through imitation by the PCD.

Speech intelligibility. A determination expressed by the speech pathologist in a percentage that deals with the degree of speech that is readily understood by the listener.

Speech screenings. Listening to speech with the intent of forming an opinion about the person's ability to speak normally. Once a determination is made, it is decided whether further evaluation is necessary.

Standardized tests. Tests that have often been used on a wide population of subjects with a compilation of normative data. People who are later tested with this instrument are compared with the normative data. Test results can be used to compare scores obtained during the initial evaluation with those compiled during the course of treatment; i.e., at the end of each treatment month. It is thought that comparing test results in this manner can give a reasonable indication of progress made in therapy.-

Stimulability testing. A method by which the speech pathologist or SM predicts the success of the PCD with any given speaking task. The SM models or says a given sound, word or phrase. If the PCD is able to repeat it accurately, the stimulability for that behavior would be noted as "good."

Stimulation. Any stimulating information or event; acts to arouse action.

Stimulated conversation. A conversation that is stimulated by the SM. It is meant to *cause* conversation, rather than allow a conversation to develop spontaneously of its own accord.

Subcortex. Any part of the brain lying below the cerebral cortex

Successive approximation. In speech therapy, a concept wherein one may need to gradually move toward the target goal, in steps, rather than accomplishing immediate mastery.

Syllable. A unit of spoken language that is larger than a speech sound, and consists of one or more vowel sounds alone, or of a consonant alone, or with one or more consonant sounds preceding or following a vowel. Examples of one syllable words: hat, ma, pa, go, yes, no; versus words of two syllables, such as fireman, bedroom, kitchen, finger, sofa.

Syntax. The orderly system or rules for combining words together in phrases or sentences to formulate thought in a specific language.

T

Telegraphic speech. Speech consisting of only certain prominent words, and lacking articles, modifiers, and other ancillary words. Telegraphic speech is the type of speech produced by people who have suffered injury to a part of the brain called Broca's area, and consists of sentences spoken in an abnormal rhythm. While people with telegraphic speech speak in meaningful but simple sentences, they omit important grammatical components. They often combine word pairs in order to convey a thought. For instance, a stroke survivor might say "sister visit" to indicate that his or her sister will be visiting. This economy of words resembles signals transmitted through a telegraph.

"Tell Me" phrases. The *Tell Me* approach is used by the SM to introduce a given word, phrase, or sentence to the PCD. The *Tell Me* word, phrase, or sentence is said with urgency to require a spoken response from the PCD.

Three-repetition model. Repeating a stimulus word numerous times by having the PCD hear, see, or say it three times.

Three-Word Level. The SM models three-word phrases and requires the PCD to respond in kind.

Time distortion. Pertains to the perceived passage of time. It is the change of perception of how fast time passes. An example in speech would be people *dancing in the conversation* and time seeming to pass very quickly.

Tolerances. To endure or accept; used in this text to refer to ascertaining what an individual with a communication difficulty (PCD) can tolerate in terms of the complexity of individual sounds, single words, phrases, or sentences when repeated after a speech model (SM). Tolerances are also observed for what an individual can comprehend from listening or reading.

Transcription. The process of writing something down, especially a conversation or speech.

Two-Word Language Formulation Model. The SM models two-word phrases for the PCD to imitate.

U

Uninhibited. Free to exhibit whatever behavior is desired without constraint.

Uvula. A small pendant-shaped fleshy lobe at the back of the soft palate.

V

Verbal mannerisms. Distinctive verbal behavioral traits or idiosyncrasies; something highly distinctive about an individual's way of speaking, setting it apart from others, such as speed, melody, or manner of talking. Traits that help one identify the speaker by the way they speak.

Verbal paraphasic errors. An error in recall in which the word desired for recall is substituted by another word which was not intended.

Verbs. Words that express action.

Visual bombardment. Presenting a word, phrase, or sentence on a computer screen or piece of paper in printed or pictorial form, and stimulating single word speaking numerous times to impress the words in printed form to the visual memory. Any word spoken repeatedly also strengthens the motor speech memory.

Vocal bombardment. The PCD's practice of saying a word, phrase, or sentence numerous times so that the motor and vocal (voice) memory can be strengthened.

Vocabulary. The sum or the stock of words used by a language, a group, or an individual.

Vowel. Speech sounds that are articulated orally and produced by the breath stream; they are not blocked or constricted by the tongue, teeth, or lips; it is the most prominent sound in the syllable, because it is voiced.

W

What It Is© Statement. Term borrowed from current language of the American culture/subculture, and coined by the author of *The Teaching of Talking*. The SM makes a statement ("I like beans."). The PCD is asked, "How about you?" The PCD models the grammar and structure of the SM's statement and responds with "I like beans."

Y

Yes/No Question. Asking a question that requires a "yes" or "no" elicits nonverbal gestures that can be readily calibrated by the SM. The *Yes/No Question* is also used in the *Teaching of Talking* method to stimulate a word, phrase, or sentence when the desired response is embedded within the question.

Bibliography

"An Overview of Aphasia; What is Aphasia?" Web MD. Accessed August 2011. http://answers.webmd.com/answers.aspx?ques=what%20is%20aphasia?

Anonymous, *Language Intervention Strategies in Adult Aphasia, 4th ed.*, (Baltimore: Lippincott Williams & Wilkins, April 15, 2001).

"Apraxia of Speech." National Institute of Health. Accessed July 2011. http://www.nidcd.gov/health/voice/apraxia.html.

"Articulatory phonetics: the study of the production of speech sounds by the articulatory and vocal tract by the speaker." Wikipedia. Accessed December 2012. http://www.en.wikipedia.org/wiki/Phonetics.

Campbell, Thomas F. "Functional Treatment Outcomes in Young Children with Motor Speech Disorders." *In Clinical Management of Motor Speech Disorders in Children*, edited by Anthony J. Caruso and Edythe A. Strand, 394. New York: Thieme Medical Publishers Inc., 1999.

Darley, Frederic L., Nancy A. Helm, Audrey Holland and Craig Linebaugh. "Techniques in Treating Mild or High-Level Aphasic Impairment." *10th Clinical Aphasiology Conference: Clinical Aphasiology Conference, June 1-5, 1980, Proceedings of the Conference.* Bar Harbor, ME: BRK Publishers, 1980. Accessed March 2011. http://aphasiology.pitt.edu/archive/00000565/.

Farlex. "Priming the Pump: A Procedure of Introducing Fluid into a Pump to Get the Water Flowing." *The Free Dictionary*. Accessed July 2011. http://thefreedictionary.com/pump+priming.

Frymark, Tobi, MA, and Carol Smith Hammond, Ph.D. "Guest Editorial: Evidence-Based Practice and Speech-Language Pathology." *Journal of Rehabilitation Research & Development. Vol. 46. no. 2.* (2009). Accessed October 2011. http://www.rehab.research.va.gov/jour/09/46/2/index.html.

"History of Lee Silverman Voice Treatment ." The National Center for Voice and Speech. Accessed November 2011. http://www.ncvs.org/research/lsvt-history.html.

Holland, Audrey L., Anita S. Halper, and Leora R. Cherney. "Tell me your story: Analysis of script topics selected by persons with aphasia." *American Journal of Speech-Language Pathology, Vol.19 198-203* (August 2010). Accessed January 2012. http://ajslp.asha.org/cgi/content/abstract/19/3/198.

Lawrence, Alex. *Looking for Success? Fight Like a Junkyard Dog.* Accessed January 20, 2012. http://www.startupflavor.com/fight-for-success/.

McCaffrey, Patrick, Ph.D. "CMSD 636 Neuro-Pathologies of Language and Cognition, Chapter 5. Aphasia-Concomitant Characteristics," The Neurosciences on the Web Series. 2011. Accessed January 2012. http://www.csuchico.edu/~pmccaffrey/syllabi/SPPA336/336unit5.html.

"Model of the World." *NLP Glossary of Terms.* Accessed February 2012. http://www.inspiritive.com.au/glossary.htm.

Molt, Lawrence, Ph.D. and J. Scott Yaruss, Ph.D. "Neurogenic Stuttering, Some Guidelines." *The Stuttering Foundation.* Accessed August 26, 2011. http://www.stutteringhelp.org/DeskLeftDefault.aspx?TabID=81.

Morales, Sarah, BS. "Stuttering or Stammering." *Children's Speech Care Center; A Division of Lynne Alba Speech Therapy, Professional Corporation.* Accessed September 2011. http://www.childspeech.net/u_iv_l.html.

"Open-Ended Questions." *Media College.* Accessed September 2011. http://www.mediacollege.com/journalism/interviews/open-ended-questions.html.

Pulvermuller, Friedemann, Ph.D., Bettina Neininger, MA, Ph.D., Thomas Elbert, Ph.D., Brigitte Rockstroh, Ph.D., Bettina Mohr, MA, Peter Koebbel, and Edward Taub, Ph.D. "Constraint-Induced Therapy of Chronic Aphasia After Stroke." *Stroke* 32 (2001): 1621. Accessed January 2012. http://stroke.ahajournals.org/content/32/7/1621.short.

Rosenbek, John C. "Speech Therapy for Apraxia: Frequency, Intensity, 1:1." *Apraxia-Kids.* 1985. Accessed March 2011. http://www.apraxia-kids.org/site/apps/nl/content3.asp?c=chKMI0PIIsE&b=788447&ct=464159.

Sackett, David. "What is Evidence-Based Practice (EBP)." *UNC Health Sciences Library,* 1996. Accessed October 2011. http://www.hsl.unc.edu/services/tutorials/ebm/whatis.htm.

Schuell, H. M., J. J. Jenkins, and E. Jiminez-Pabon, *Aphasia in Adults* (New York, NY: Harper and Row, 1964). H. M. Schuell, V. Carroll, and B. S. Street, "Clinical Treatment of Aphasia," *Journal of Speech and Hearing Disorders,* 1955. C. M. Scott, Editor's Note, Journal of Speech and Hearing Disorders.

Schuell, Hildred, James J. Jenkins, Edward Jiménez-Pabón. *Aphasia in Adults: Diagnosis, Prognosis, and Treatment, 4th ed.* (Hoeber Medical Division, Harper & Row, 1969).

Sims Wyeth & Co. "Communication Skills: Presence in Conversation." *High Stakes Presentations.* Accessed September 25, 2009. http://www.simswyeth. com/20090925-communication-skills-presence-in-conversation/.

"Speech and Language Developmental Milestones." *National Institute on Deafness and Other Communication Disorders, National Institutes of Health.* Updated September 2010. Accessed March, 2011. http://www.nidcd.nih.gov/health/ voice/pages/speechandlanguage.aspx.

"Speech Language Assessment; Target: Texas Guide for Effective Teaching; Speech Language Assessment; Texas Statement Leadership for Autism Training." March 2009. Accessed January 2011. http://www.txautism.net/docs/Guide/ Evaluation/SpeechLanguage.pdf.

Starch, Sandy A. and Robert C. Marshall. "Who's on First? A Treatment Approach for Name Recall with Aphasic Patients." *In Clinical Aphasiology Conference: 16ᵗʰ Clinical Aphasiology Conference.* Minneapolis, MN: BRK Publishers, 73-79. June 8-12, 1986. Accessed March 2011. http://aphasiology.pitt.edu/ archive/00000895/.

"The 'Good Life'." *Happiness:Eudaimonia; Thoughts from Different Traditions.* Accessed November 2011. http://doggo.tripod.com/dogggoodlife.html.

VanRiper, Charles, Ph.D. *Speech Correction, Principle and Methods* 6ᵗʰ ed. Englewood Cliffs, NJ 07632: Prentice-Hall, Inc., 1978.

—. *Speech Correction, Principles and Methods.* 3ʳᵈ ed. Englewood Cliffs, NJ: Prentice-Hall, Inc., 1954.

Vinson, Betsy Partin. *Essentials for Speech-Language Pathologists.* San Diego, CA: Singular Publishing Group, 2001.

Wepman, Joseph M. *Recovery from Aphasia.* New York: Ronald Press, 1951.

Wikipedia. "Pedagogy." Accessed November 2010. http://www.wikipedia.org/ pedagogy

Zareva, Alla, Ph.D. "Frontier Words in the L2 Mental Lexicon." *Ohio University Working Papers in Applied Linguistics: 2008 Volume.* 2008. Accessed March 2011. http://www.ohiou.edu/linguistics/workingpapers/2008/zareva_2008. html.

Printed in the USA
CPSIA information can be obtained
at www.ICGtesting.com
LVHW041212210924
791747LV00002B/140